DEMENTIA

The Journey Ahead

DEMENTIA

The Journey Ahead

A PRACTICAL GUIDE *for*
IN-HOME CAREGIVERS

SUSAN KISER SCARFF

ANN KISER ZULTNER

LANGDON STREET PRESS

Langdon Street Press
212 3rd Avenue North, Suite 290
Minneapolis, MN 55401
612.455.2293
www.langdonstreetpress.com

ISBN-13: 978-1-936782-95-6
LCCN: 2012933167

Distributed by Itasca Books

All Photos Courtesy of the Author.

Printed in the United States of America

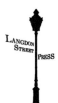

LANGDON
STREET PRESS

DISCLAIMER

I do not have a medical background. I earned my diploma as a caregiver by misfortune, experience, and research. After numerous doctors' appointments ending in frustration, Red was accurately diagnosed by Dr. Bruce Miller at the University of San Francisco, with Primary Progressive Aphasia (PPA), a form of frontotemporal dementia (FTD). There is no cure for dementia, and pharmaceutical treatments to help control symptoms and behavioral issues are limited in what they can accomplish.

The information in this handbook may not be suitable for all dementia patients and caregivers. Each caregiver should make an informed choice in conjunction with his or her physician.

ACKNOWLEDGMENTS

I am eternally grateful to my idol Harv and my Yahoo! online PPA support group; Dr. Bruce Miller; Dr. Gary Grove; Dr. Linda Hon; Michelle and Martin Trump, Jr.; Kris Young; Diana Ing; Denise Boyd; and Hospice of the Valley. I could not have successfully accomplished my mission without your years of devotion, kindness, companionship, patience, knowledge, and laughter.

My special thanks to my online fellow caregiver and cohort in crime, Virginia Pasquarelli. She encouraged my literary endeavor with humor, and recommended book titles such as *Susie and What She Learned About Poop,* and *My Husband Keeps Peeing in the Flower Pot: Can Anyone Tell Me What to Do?* In the midst of her own personal turmoil, Ginny recorded her deepest thoughts and feelings, composing many heartfelt poems that I am honored to include in this book. Ginny's mother, Virginia, lost her battle with dementia on August 8, 2011.

DEDICATION

According to the Alzheimer's Association in 2011, "Dementia impacts 15 million unpaid caregivers in the United States."

This book is dedicated to the unpaid dementia caregivers who find themselves in the unenviable position of caring for a loved one diagnosed with dementia.

My husband, Red, proved to me that patience is a prerequisite, laughter is the best medicine, and a smile is worth a thousand words.

AUTHOR'S NOTE

Red was born April 25, 1933 in Greenville, Michigan. He graduated from high school in 1951 as a state football icon. Granted a full track and football scholarship, Red attended the University of Colorado in Boulder, where he was a member of the Delta Tau Delta Fraternity and the ROTC program.

Red graduated in 1955 with a Bachelor of Science degree in Geology and Mineralogy. After college, Red enlisted and served in the US Air Force as a fighter pilot, flying F-100s from 1955 to 1959. In 1957, while stationed at Nellis Air Force Base in Nevada, he participated in air operations atmospheric thermonuclear testing. He was then off to Bitburg, Germany for two years, where he flew F-100s and sampled beer. As a Captain in the Air Force Reserves, "The Red Baron" was given an honorable discharge in 1967.

Between his commitments to the Air Force, he attended graduate school at UCLA and earned an MBA. He lived and worked all over the world in various capacities, eventually establishing his own consulting and partnership investing corporation in

1983. Red fulfilled his competitive spirit and need for freedom as an athlete, avid sailor, and a commercial sailplane pilot until his diagnosis in 1997.

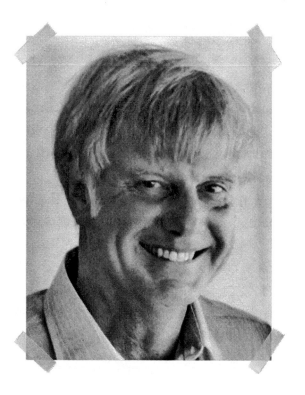

Harold Maxwell Scarff, Jr., aka Red, 1933-2006
Photograph taken October 15, 1982

CONTENTS

A PRAYER FOR THE CAREGIVER
Bruce McIntyre

Unknown and often unnoticed,
you are a hero nonetheless.

For your love, sacrificial, is God at his best.

You walk by faith in the darkness
of the great unknown,
and your courage, even in weakness,
gives life to your beloved.

You hold shaking hands and
provide the ultimate care:
Your presence, the knowing,
that you are simply there.

You rise to face the giant of disease and despair;
it is your finest hour, though you may be unaware.

You are resilient, amazing, and beauty unexcelled,
you are the caregiver and you have done well!

INTRODUCTION

"There are only four kinds of people in the world—
those who have been caregivers,
those who currently are caregivers,
those who will be caregivers,
and those who need caregivers."
—Rosalynn Carter

Today, an estimated 5.4 million Americans have Alzheimer's disease or a related neurodegenerative disease; many live with the disease for 20 years before symptoms are diagnosed. Research into the underlying causes of these disorders and in developing treatments is surging ahead, giving us great hope for the future. But what about the family members caring for patients now? What can be done for them?

Caregiving can be a scary, challenging, and wonderful experience. It is a skill that must be learned over time; it is not something that most of us know instinctively. I met Susan Scarff while caring for her husband. From the moment I met her I knew that she was special and would use the catastrophe that had afflicted Red to do something good. In this remarkable book, Susan tells the loving story of living with and caring for her husband as he fell victim to primary progressive aphasia. She speaks of her experience caring for Red so that others can learn. It is Susan's gift back to us.

As she describes, in the beginning there are important plans to be made and put in place: preparing for medical, legal, and financial contingencies; developing a support network; getting organized. Caregivers often need a reminder to take care of themselves so that they can continue to care for their loved one. Then there are the practical issues of dealing with a relentlessly degenerative disease that includes some very difficult behaviors as well as decreasing ability to function in their daily lives. Finally, grief is an important part of being a caregiver. Finding the right expression for it is an essential part of self-care. This practical, realistic guide walks us through all these phases.

Caregivers make an incredible contribution not only to the lives of their loved ones, but also to our society as a whole. The journey caregivers embark on is one of the most difficult journeys in life: the road is hard, and they are expected to endure physical, emotional, and psychological hardships along the way. I hope this guide inspires you to take advantage of the help and support available to you. There are numerous services offered by the professional health care community. The wider community of caregivers and the patient's loved ones is large and welcoming. You are not alone in this. Caregiving touches all of us in some way.

Dr. Bruce L. Miller
UCSF Memory and Aging Center
April 2011

PROLOGUE

My husband disguised it well, but I knew.

I had known for the last seven or eight years. He was sixty-five and I was forty-seven. We had been married for sixteen years. The eighteen years between us never made a difference. His sense of humor, wit, intelligence, and gift of gab were incomparable, his laughter contagious. He was a knight in shining armor for me and for his family. He had always surpassed me mentally and physically. Until now.

In 1991, my husband was demoted, without notice or explanation, from his new position as president of a furniture company that spans three states. Within one month of the demotion, he quit the furniture company and took a job in airborne laser mapping. The new job required him to commute out-of-state during the week and fly home on the weekends.

One weekend, without warning, Red could not remember our home address. His short-term memory loss was obvious, and his grammar and comprehension were declining. Weeping like a baby, he declared, "Something is wrong with my brain."

In the mid 1990s, Red was screened for Alzheimer's disease. The screening amounted to no more than a short mathematical and verbal memory assessment. As far as his primary care physician was concerned, he passed with flying colors. I vocally rejected his doctor's opinion, but to no avail. Aw shucks, I'm just the little missus. What do I know?

As the days turned to months, months into years, his good judgment waned and he became socially uninhibited. I would come home from work to find complete strangers on a tour of our home, chatting with Red over tea and crumpets. He would carry our financial portfolio with him in a briefcase for show and tell. He would fixate on bald gentlemen, point and laugh. Spitting and passing gas in stores became a daily, exhilarating event for him. Red would no longer urinate in the toilet, only a sink. I once caught him drinking water teaspoon by teaspoon from the kitchen faucet.

For two years, all he ate was store-bought fried chicken. He forgot the names of familiar objects and people. Was I imagining this? My husband of sixteen years was acting out like a three-year-old. Red was scared and confused. In lucid moments, he talked of committing suicide.

On October 13, 1998, my fear was realized. After days of testing at the Mayo Clinic, our lives went to hell with the diagnosis of one word: dementia. I had a clinical diagnosis and MRI to back up what I had known for years. With the doctor's declaration, I launched into profanity. I suppose it would have been more tasteful to sit silently and weep. Truth be told, I envisioned turning over office furniture and throwing every chair in the room out the window. That might have been in bad taste, but I would have felt better. The diagnosis did not faze my husband.

During the next few days, I wrapped my brain around what the future had in store for us and briefly considered turning to alcohol. I was now a statistic and my husband's principal advocate. Our journey into the unknown was underway.

Within a year of my husband's diagnosis, I became a poster child for caregiver burnout. My tolerance at home and work had diminished. I was devoted to my job of ten years at the Desert Botanical Garden, but it was obvious to me that it was time to move on. The staff and volunteers had no idea what I was going through at home, and I was not willing to share for fear of making it an excuse for my behavior. It was not their problem. I was short-tempered, absentminded, tired—but never late. I would not survive working with the public and volunteers by day and caregiving for a dementia patient at night. The role of fecal and fecal fumes manager on the home front was enough to cope with.

All at once, our world became very small, and we were trapped inside our own private prison. I had lost my partner and misplaced myself. Becoming the boss of both our lives was not a role I would have chosen to play.

Dementia is a long-term life-altering disorder that one cannot endure alone. Could I make the most of what we had and employ my questions, mistakes, and successes as a teaching aid for myself and others? My husband was counting on me, and my own sanity depended on it.

As a caregiver, your personal time is very limited. How are you going to become your patient's protector if you have no experience, time, or resources available? This text is a user-friendly guide for the long journey ahead, designed to help you choose your battles, plan for the future, and become proactive in the health and well-being of your loved one. It also includes the visual evolution of a dementia patient— my husband, Red. The images of my husband are meant to educate, not shock and embarrass.

Current statistics indicate there are as many as six to eight million people in the United States and potentially thirty-five million in the world suffering from dementia. These are astonishing figures. Even more astonishing? Experts predict these numbers will continue to double every twenty years, unless we have some significant medical breakthroughs in dementia prevention and treatment.

LOVE
Virginia Pasquarelli

Dementia is an ugly word.
We don't know much
about what's ahead,
but we know to fear it.

I love him.
He's a burden.
I gladly and lovingly carry it.
I carry him.

I lean in close,
feel his warmth.
He's somewhere, and he's here.
He's alive.

The love is what
gets me through.
It's what I think of
when we are restless at night.

It doesn't get easier.
He doesn't get better.
But I try.
And the love gets us through.

CHAPTER ONE

The Diagnosis

Dementia is a progressive, incurable group of symptoms that affects memory, behavior, reasoning, learning, communication, and daily functioning. Dementia may be caused by a number of degenerative neurological disorders as well as clinical syndromes such as Alzheimer's disease, Vascular dementia, Lewy body disease, Pick's disease, Frontotemporal dementia (FTD), Corticobasal degeneration, Huntington's disease, Creutzfeldt-Jakob disease, and Parkinson's dementia. To date, an accurate diagnosis can only be confirmed with a brain autopsy.

Early signs of dementia are usually noticed by family and friends of the patient; communicating your observations to your physicians will alert them of the need for further evaluation.

SYMPTOMS

The following list is a specialized range of symptoms that will be useful as you prepare your observations and concerns for your doctor's appointment:

- Progressive memory loss
- An inability to concentrate
- A decrease in problem-solving and judgment capabilities
- Confusion
- Hallucinations and delusions
- Altered sensation or perception
- Agnosia: Impaired recognition of objects, people, and/or senses
- Altered sleep patterns
- Motor system impairment
  - Apraxia: Impaired skilled motor function
    - Inability to reproduce numerical figures
    - Inability to mimic hand positions
    - Inability to get dressed
  - Gait changes
  - Inappropriate movements
- Disorientation
  - Person, place, time disorientation
  - Visual-spatial disorientation
  - Inability to interpret environmental cues
- Specific disorders of problem-solving or learning

- o   Inability to generalize
- o   Loss of abstract thinking
- o   Impaired calculating ability
- o   Inability to learn
- Memory deficit
  - o   Short-term memory problems
  - o   Long-term memory problems
- Aphasia, or impaired language ability
  - o   Inability to comprehend speech
  - o   Inability to read
  - o   Inability to write
  - o   Inability to speak
  - o   Inability to form words
  - o   Inability to name objects
  - o   Poor enunciation
  - o   Inappropriate speech; inappropriate language or verbal gibberish
  - o   Inability to repeat a phrase; alternatively, the persistent repetition of phrases
- Personality changes
  - o   Irritability
  - o   Weak temper control
  - o   Anxiety
  - o   Depression
  - o   Indecisiveness
  - o   Self-centeredness
  - o   Inflexibility
  - o   No observable mood (flat affect)

- o Inappropriate mood or behavior
- o Withdrawal from social interaction
- o Inability to function or interact in social or personal situations
- o Inability to maintain employment
- o Decreased ability to care for oneself
- o Decreased interest in daily living activities
- o Lack of spontaneity

Additional symptoms associated with the late stage of this disease:
- Difficulty swallowing
- Incontinence

As the primary caregiver, prioritize your objectives following the initial diagnosis with a to-do list resembling the one below:

1. Get a second opinion.
2. Create a support system.
3. Make sure finances and legal documents are in order.
4. Be prepared: Assemble a personal portfolio.
5. Take care of yourself.

GET A SECOND OPINION

One opinion is never enough. Many primary care physicians are not trained to identify neurological disorders and syndromes. Frequently, they bandage the symptoms with medication, or misdiagnose the condition altogether. Your mission should be to obtain a valid medical diagnosis from a neurologist. As his or her advocate, your loved one is depending on you. An accurate diagnosis is essential so you can both begin to plan for your future.

DAILY JOURNAL

Creating a written record of your loved one's activities, abnormalities, and indiscretions is an excellent way to communicate with physicians and family members. A written record will help facilitate a more accurate diagnosis, and eliminates the difficult chore of remembering all that has transpired. Keeping a journal has the added benefit of reducing caregiver stress. Your daily journal should include the following information about the patient:

- Medications
- Allergies
- Memory Status
- Daily Activities
- Behavior
- Eating Habits and Cravings
- Appearance
- Unusual Events
- Sleep Routine
- Questions

As they say, a picture is worth a thousand words. You may want to consider videotaping or photographing your loved one as a physical reference for the physician and yourself. Keeping a record of your loved one's progression will likely expedite a diagnosis.

THE WHO'S WHO OF DOCTORS

The following doctors will play an integral role in your new life as a caregiver:

Family Practitioner / General Practitioner

The family practitioner (FP) and the general practitioner (GP) are physicians whose practices are not oriented toward a specific medical specialty, but instead cover a variety of medical problems in patients of all ages. Many managed care insurance plans use these doctors as "gatekeepers" to coordinate health care benefits and control costs. Your family practitioner or general practitioner (also known as your primary care physician) will be the doctor who refers you to a neurologist.

Neurologist

A neurologist is a medical doctor who diagnoses and treats disorders of the nervous system, brain, and spinal cord. The neurologist will likely be the specialist who provides you with a definitive diagnosis.

Geriatric Psychiatrist

A geriatric psychiatrist is a medical doctor who diagnoses and treats mental and emotional disorders in the elderly. If appropriate, a geriatric psychiatrist will prescribe medications to help control the progression of the disease and its associated behaviors.

Neuropsychologist

A neuropsychologist is a professional psychologist who has earned a Ph.D. (rather than an M.D.) and specializes in the relationship between the nervous system—especially the brain—and the cerebral or mental functions such as language, memory, and perception. A neuropsychologist will conduct numerous tests to evaluate a patient's level of impairment.

Our neuropsychologist helped share my burden. She provided me with recommendations regarding level of patient care, stage-appropriate patient supervision, further patient evaluation, necessary changes in my husband's home environment, nutrition, what to expect and how to cope emotionally as the dementia progressed, and how to best care for my husband and myself.

It may be difficult to leave your home to visit a doctor's office. If so, the Alzheimer's Association may be able to provide you with a recommendation for a neuropsychologist who will come to your home. Medicare covered most of the cost for us.

CREATE A SUPPORT SYSTEM

Contact the Alzheimer's Association after the formal diagnosis. Their 24-hour helpline number is 1-800-272-3900 and their website is located at http://www.alz.org. This organization has programs and services available in most areas of the United States, and is willing and able to help with any questions or concerns you or the patient may have. If they can't answer a question, they will refer you to additional resources.

Join a Support Group

It is important to connect with individuals who have been in your situation or are currently going through the same experience. Start by asking the Alzheimer's Association for contact information for support groups that meet in your area. If you are lucky, your local Alzheimer's chapter may have their support groups organized by age or diagnosis. To gain the full benefit, join a group with similar needs and interests to your own.

The Internet is also a good resource for locating support groups. Online support groups are usually specialized, organized, and managed by members going through the same kinds of experiences. Yahoo! Support Groups are a great place to start. You can find a directory of them here: http://groups.yahoo.com.

Contact one or more of the following professional caregiving resources for additional information and support.

The National Association of Area Agencies on Aging

http://www.n4a.org

Phone Number: 1-202-872-8888

In most cities, your local chapter of the Area Agencies on Aging is listed in the phone book.

Eldercare Locator

http://www.eldercare.gov/Eldercare/Public/Home.asp

Toll-Free Phone Number: 1-800-677-1116

Family Caregiver Alliance

http://www.caregiver.org

Toll-Free Phone Number: 1-800-445-8106

Today's Caregiver Magazine

http://www.caregiver.com

Toll-Free Phone Number: 1-800-829-2734

National Family Caregivers Association (NFCA)
http://www.nfcacares.org
The NFCA site also features its own resource list, which can be found here:
http://www.thefamilycaregiver.org/ed/resources.cfm
Toll-Free Phone Number: 1-800-896-3650

The Association for Frontotemporal Dementias
http://ftd-picks.org
Toll-Free Phone Number: 1-866-507-7222

Northwestern University
http://www.brain.northwestern.edu

Additional caregiving resources can be found in Appendix C.

In addition to these professional resources, enlist the help of family, friends, church leaders, physicians, senior centers, and volunteer groups.

Negative or unconstructive family interactions can have a traumatic emotional impact on caregivers. Some family members may be in denial of the diagnosis or disagree about the care and management of their loved one, creating unnecessary family conflict. It will take time for everyone to make the emotional adjustment. Initially, everyone will have an opinion on the care of your loved one. Long distance family members in particular should not assume they know what goes on in a typical day.

As challenging as it may seem under these circumstances, the elected caregiver must share the burden with other family members, if only for his or her own well-being. Dementia is devastating for everyone involved. As a family, strive to achieve unified team work, effective communication, and ongoing support for the caregiver and patient.

THE ORGANIZATION AND MAINTENANCE OF LEGAL DOCUMENTS AND FINANCES

Engage the services of an elder law attorney, preferably one who specializes in dementia. Do NOT go to the phone book to find an attorney! You are at your most vulnerable, and "professionals" with questionable backgrounds are just waiting to take advantage of you. If possible, always get a recommendation from a family member or trusted friend first. If this is not possible, the Alzheimer's Association or your local Area Agency on Aging can provide you with the names of elder law attorneys in your area. Because dementia is a progressive disease, it is imperative that you have the proper documents in place and signed as soon as possible. A dementia patient must be of reasonable sound mind, understand what he or she is signing, and be able to sign his or her name on all official documentation. As the disease progresses, the patient will no longer be able to manage his or her legal or financial affairs. If your legal documents were prepared and signed before the diagnosis, make sure you store them in a safe place and keep them up-to-date.

LEGAL DOCUMENTS

In order to complete the following legal documents, you may require professional assistance from an elder law attorney. The caregiver, trusted family member, attorney, and the doctor should each have copies of all legal documents.

Financial Durable Power of Attorney

This legal document allows the person with dementia (known as "the principal") to name a person (called "an agent," and typically a trusted family member or friend) who is responsible for making financial decisions when he or she is no longer able; in other words, when the patient has become legally incompetent. Most powers of attorney are "durable," meaning they are valid even after the principal can no longer make decisions for himself or herself.

Health Care/Medical Durable Power of Attorney

This legal document allows a person to name an individual ("the agent") to act on his or her behalf to make health care decisions when he or she is no longer able. These decisions include choosing health care providers, treatments, and care facilities. Arrange for a HIPAA Release Authority to be added to your health care power of attorney documents. This allows you or your agent to obtain the patient's health information and medical records. This is crucial if your loved one loses the ability to comprehend or communicate in the latter stage of dementia.

Be aware that laws in reference to advance directives such as a DNR (do not resuscitate) vary from state to state. You may want to check with your local Alzheimer's Association and/or attorney for further information.

Living Will

A Living Will documents an individual's choices for future medical decisions, such as the use of artificial life support. A Living Will only comes into play when a doctor decides that the person is irreversibly ill or critically injured and near death.

Will

A Will legally documents who the person with dementia has chosen as the executor (in other words, the person who will manage the estate) as well as defines the individuals who will receive the estate ("the beneficiaries"). A Will only takes effect when the person with dementia dies.

Living Trust

A Living Trust is created by a live person[s] capable of making his or her own financial decisions. The person can appoint a responsible individual of his or her choosing (usually a trusted family member) as trustee to carefully invest and manage the property and assets of the trust during the patient's life, or after his or her passing.

It is very important that you become familiar with the legal definitions of the following terms:

Guardianship

When a person is appointed Guardianship by the court, that person has the legal responsibility and authority to make decisions and manage the patient's finances, health care, and safety. A legal guardian is under the supervision of the court; in some states, the guardian is required to appear annually in front of a judge to give periodic reports about the status of the patient (or "ward") and the estate. In Arizona, petitioning for Conservatorship is redundant if you already have Guardianship. Legal Guardianship defines and permits all of the legal requirements necessary for a caregiver to avoid spending more money obtaining a Conservatorship. Please check with a trusted attorney before investing your time and money obtaining any unnecessary legal documents. Legal obligations and definitions vary from state to state. Guardianship and Conservatorship parameters may overlap.

Conservator

A conservator is an individual appointed by the court, legally responsible for safeguarding and managing the estate and financial affairs of a person suffering from physical or mental limitations. In some states, the conservator not only manages the financial affairs, or "estate," but also "oversees the conservatee's daily decisions such as health care or living arrangements. The process requires a relative or friend to petition the local superior court for appointment of a specific conservator, with written notice served on the potential conservatee. The conservator may be removed by order of the court if no longer needed, or for failure to perform his or her duties."

INSURANCE

Once a diagnosis of dementia has been established, it is typically no longer possible for patients to obtain many—if any—types of insurance. As a result, it is imperative that you become familiar with the following types of insurance.

Medicare

Medicare is a federal health insurance program for people ages 65 and older. Medicare covers inpatient hospital care, a percentage of doctors' fees, a percentage of medical items, and outpatient prescription drugs. Under certain conditions, the program also provides some home health care, including skilled nursing care and rehabilitation therapy. It does not pay for long-term nursing home care.

Medigap

Medigap insurance fills gaps in Medicare coverage. The more expensive Medigap insurance policies (also called "Medicare Supplement Insurance") may cover additional items.

Medicaid

Medicaid pays for the medical care of people with very low income and asset levels. Under most circumstances, this program also pays for the long-term care of those whose finances have been depleted. Sufferers of dementia should use caution when giving away assets to family members in order to qualify for Medicaid. Talk to an elder law attorney before making any significant financial arrangement.

Disability insurance

Disability insurance provides income for employees who are no longer capable of working due to illness or injury. An employer-paid disability policy can replace a percentage of a person's gross income.

Long-term care insurance

Long-term care insurance typically pays for the costs of most care settings, including nursing homes. If the person with dementia has a long-term care policy, carefully review the material to confirm whether dementia is covered, when the patient can begin receiving benefits, and what kind of care the policy covers.

Life insurance

Life insurance can be a valuable source of cash. The person with dementia may be able to receive a part of the policy's face value as a loan, known as a viatical loan, paid off upon the person's death. Some life insurance companies will allow a terminally ill patient to receive a portion of the insurance money prior to death if you add a living benefit or purchase an "accelerated" death benefit.

FINANCES

A diagnosis of dementia inevitably leads to many expenses you as the caregiver may not have considered. Probable future expenses include:

- Medical treatment/lab work
- Prescription drugs for you and your loved one
- Personal care supplies such as diapers
- Temporary respite care services provided outside the home
- Adult daycare services

- In-home care services
- Assisted living and nursing home care

Caring for a dementia patient is very expensive. The last two years of my husband's life I spent between $6,000 and $10,000 a month out-of-pocket providing for his special needs. My expenses were substantially reduced when Hospice stepped in.

You may be able to obtain financial assistance from one or more of the following sources:

Social Security Disability Income

Social Security Disability Income is for workers younger than 65 who qualify for benefits. To qualify, the person must meet the Social Security Administration's definition of disability. Generally, that means proving that the person with dementia is unable to work in any occupation and that the condition will either last at least a year or is expected to result in death.

For more information about federal programs for people with disabilities, visit the Social Security Administration's website at http://www.ssa.gov/disability, call your local social security office, or call the Social Security Administration toll-free at 1-800-772-1213.

Taxes

As a caregiver, consult a tax professional to find out what deductions you are eligible to claim. Medical expenses used to improve or avoid mental or physical illnesses usually qualify.

Veteran's Benefits

The United States Department of Veterans Affairs (VA) is responsible for administering programs associated with veterans' benefits for veterans, their families, and survivors.

Go to http://www.va.gov/health for information on eligibility and benefits, and to search for answers to frequently asked questions. You can also call the Veterans Administration toll-free number at 1-800-827-1000. Their goal is to respond to inquiries within five business days.

Retirement Savings

Retirement savings include individual retirement accounts (IRAs) and employee-funded retirement plans, such as a 401(k) and 403(b).

Personal Savings and Assets

Personal savings and assets include stocks, bonds, savings accounts, real estate, and any valuable personal property such as jewelry or artwork.

BE PREPARED
Create a Portfolio

Our most indispensable reference was a notebook

I put together and labeled "Our Portfolio." It was an all-in-one database of our personal and financial lives. When talking with our accountant, attorneys, doctors, or simply trying to plan for the future, I was able to access all of the required information from one location. A copy of our portfolio was kept in a fireproof safe and a copy was mailed to my sister in case of an emergency. Being organized will save you a lot of time and aggravation.

Essential Items To Include in Your Portfolio
- Driver's license and license plate numbers
- Pertinent phone numbers
- Veteran's discharge papers
- Duplicate marriage license
- Alarm system passwords
- Copy of birth certificate
- Social Security number
- Passport
- Emergency contact information
- Support group contact information
- Personal physicians' contact information
- Insurance policy numbers, annual costs, date last paid
- Copy of Medicare and insurance cards
- A record of monthly income
- Bank account numbers and amounts
- Monthly expense spreadsheets

- Retirement account information, including names and numbers
- Financial consultant contact information
- The location of any safety deposit boxes and cosigners
- House deeds
- Car titles
- Vehicle Identification Number
- Inventory of collectibles
- Financial misc./other assets
- Superior Court Guardianship documents

Create a health records emergency kit, or a smaller version of the portfolio, by compiling all of your loved one's health care records in one location, such as a folder or three-ring binder. You may need immediate access to this information if you unexpectedly have to call the paramedics or visit the emergency room. Information to keep in your emergency kit includes:

- List of known allergies
- Current medications, dosage, and prescribing doctor
- Pharmacy phone numbers
- Diagnosis on physician's letterhead
- Primary care doctor's name and phone number
- Neurologist's name and phone number
- Geriatric Psychiatrist's name and phone number

- Emergency contact information
- Copy of insurance cards
- Copy of legal guardianship/conservator papers
- Copy of Health Care Power of Attorney with HIPAA Release Authority
- Copy of Living Will
- Photo I.D./driver's license
- Caregivers' contact information
- Medical Release Form
- If desired, a Do Not Resuscitate (DNR) order

A Medical Release Form asserts the caregiver's authorization to release the patient's medical records from the patient's primary physician to an attending physician in the emergency room or newly acquired symptom-specific physicians.

Refer to Appendix B for copies of the sample
Health Records Emergency Kit and Medical Release Form.

Sample Emergency Names and Numbers Card

Following is a sample Emergency Names and Numbers Card. This is a business card size document that lists important names and phone numbers. It is easy to carry and should be included in your emergency kit, your wallet, and the wallets of your loved ones. Make several copies that can be handed to emergency room staff to save time. Produce them on your own or enlist a business card company to print them for you.

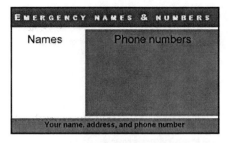

Front side of sample
business size emergency card

Red Scarff Medications/2006
Red's meds
• *Abilify* : 15mgs-AM
• *Tylenol:* 1/2-1 Tbs. daily
• **Depakene: 2 teas AM**
Allergies: sulfa drugs
ativan

Backside of sample
business size emergency card

You may also want to keep your emergency phone numbers in a larger format next to your home telephone for easy access.

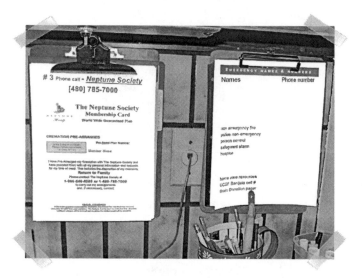

Enlarged emergency card phone numbers
by the phone

I cannot stress enough how important it is to be proactive and prepared for the worst. On my own emergency contact card, I included telephone numbers for the following contacts:

- Primary physicians
- Family members
- Attorney
- Home care resources
- Poison Control
- Non-emergency fire department
- Hospice
- Brain donation

Erasable Calendar

Another great way to stay organized is by using a magnetic erasable calendar. These calendars are available at most major retail stores. Attach the calendar to the refrigerator or next to the telephone and use it to keep track of both of your schedules. You can also use it to track your loved one's progression by documenting variables like weight, bowel movements, and temperature.

For about one year, Red kept track of the days by crossing them off the calendar. It seemed to give him a sense of control, confidence, and order.

Picture ID

Obtain a photo identification card from the Department of Motor Vehicles, or create a photo ID on your computer. Put several copies of the ID in your wallet and in your loved one's wallet. This is important to have if your loved one becomes disoriented or confrontational with a stranger or police officer, or if he or she wanders off and gets lost. The card is actually the size of a business card.

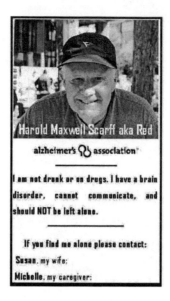

Computer-generated photo ID

MedicAlert + Safe Return Program
Enroll in the latest MedicAlert + Alzheimer's Association Safe Return Program. This new program provides 24-hour emergency response for wandering patients, medical emergencies, family notification, and care consultation. You can call the toll-free number, 1-888-572-8566, to receive a member enrollment application, or find more information at http://www.medicalert.org/safereturn.

MY EXPERIENCE
I searched for answers and a referral to a neurologist for over five years before receiving my husband's

first diagnosis of dementia: Pick's disease, a degenerative, incurable loss of brain function. After overcoming the shock and denial, we decided to get a second opinion from the University of California, San Francisco Memory and Aging Center. Red was put through days of testing, physically and mentally. Ultimately, same outcome, different brand name.

Diagnosis: Primary Progressive Aphasia (PPA), a form of Frontotemporal Dementia

Prognosis: progressive and incurable

Prior to being diagnosed, my husband wrote the following list for me to give to the plumber. This list helped to substantiate his physician's diagnosis of Primary Progressive Aphasia (PPA).

Red's List for the plumber

1) they tid te rewrite we do enny the the fes we prot? to
2) Jron to mor the stuff - he hip me put the dor
3) Tho Rig the stugy — put scom greaue the less he hass
4) whe he can come over hear —
4) We can provide the stuffe to thus he hass
3) we will proffitbe the
7) he aah the gloident

Should you tell your loved one that his or her initial diagnosis will eventually turn into dementia? I think the answer to this question must be considered on a case-by-case basis. I chose not to go into great detail with my spouse. That only would have made matters worse for him. In our situation, my husband's first neurologist gave us a full ten minutes of his valuable time to present us with a life-altering diagnosis. During our conversation, the doctor instructed me to have Red's driver's and pilot's licenses permanently revoked. He then handed me some pamphlets to read in reference to the Safe Return Program and recommended I sign him up immediately and seek counseling. We were escorted out the door in a stupor, left to our thoughts of what the future would bring. Oh my God, where do I start?

I paid close attention to Red's reaction and was surprised to observe his immediate relief. For the last five or six years, he had seen himself as a failure. He was depressed and sometimes talked of suicide. Now he had an explanation that he would, thankfully, never fully comprehend. That was a blessing.

At the time of diagnosis, Red's language and comprehension skills were already severely compromised; mercifully, he did not understand the gravity of his doctor's analysis. Occasionally, he would ask me why he could not "think right." I would tell him he had a problem with his memory and leave it at that.

While we were searching for an accurate diagnosis, our family practitioner attempted to treat my husband's agitation and behavioral issues with a drug called Ativan. Ativan, which goes by the generic name of Lorazapam, is an anti-anxiety drug used for the management of anxiety disorders associated with depression. Our physician was not aware that many dementia patients have an unfavorable response when given this medication. For this reason, avoid medications such as Valium, Xanax, and Ativan if you suspect a diagnosis of dementia, as they may create more problems than they solve.

A couple of years after my husband's diagnosis, I quit my job to begin a new career as caregiver. For ten years, my job as staff member and volunteer at the Desert Botanical Garden had been a significant part of my identity and social circle. Overnight, I felt isolated, alienated not only from my friends and family, but from the world as well. My family lived in another state and our friends appeared to fear the diagnosis, consequently disappearing one by one. Life as I knew it had ended. I needed emotional support and finally realized that no one was going to volunteer to provide it—it was up to me to get what I so desperately required, and that was help, in every sense of the word.

At my lowest point, I contacted the Alzheimer's Helpline. I needed to whine and snivel to someone who was or had been in my position. The volunteer patiently spoke with me about our shared experiences and gave me a referral to an elder law attorney and a wonderful neuropsychologist.

Our neuropsychologist made weekly visits to our home. This young Ph.D. was the first person to become a part of my small, but invaluable, support system. We discussed emotional and behavioral issues my husband and I were encountering, and she educated me on what to expect as Red's dementia progressed. She customized our meetings, focusing on issues we would be faced with in the near future, solutions to these problems, and caregiver coping skills. Since my husband was over 65, Medicare paid the bill. The counseling was priceless and pointed me in the right direction. Our neuropsychologist was our therapist, crisis manager, constant resource, and intervention director. I would have ended up in a sanitarium without her support. My advice to you is to find an experienced dementia neuropsychologist, geriatric psychiatrist, or social worker who meets your specific needs as a caregiver. Make an effort to schedule weekly or bi-monthly appointments with that person. His or her advice and support will be invaluable.

My first and last in-person support group met once a month at the local senior center. At the time, I was in my forties. The group was comprised of spouses of Alzheimer's patients between the ages of forty and sixty. I managed to attend group meetings for several months, scared to death something horrendous would happen to Red while I was away from home. Ultimately, there was no similarity between my husband's symptomology and the rest of the group. It left me frustrated, angry, scared, lost, and back to square one. I needed answers and positive reinforcement, not the name of the last caregiver who died due to years of stress. Given how many varieties of support are out there, I should not have let this deter me. The key is to find whatever method of support best fits your needs.

My online support group turned out to be the most educational, encouraging, and empathetic of any of my resources. I will never forget these wonderful people. To this day, we are still going through hell and back together.

When friends and family learned of my husband's diagnosis, I heard many people say, "I wish there was something I could do," or, "Call me if you need help." In retrospect, I should have had a list ready with dates, times, places, and needs like a cooked dinner, a grocery run, or housekeeping. In my experience, if you don't jump at the opportunity for help, most people run in the opposite direction.

Unfortunately, because I did not want to burden my family or friends, we were isolated. I would often think, *What the heck am I going to talk about at lunch with the girls when my life revolves around my spouse's next bowel movement?* Caregiving is alienating. Make the most of the support and resources at hand, so you have enough energy left to be proactive and assertive on behalf of your loved one.

Desperate for answers and respite, I admitted my husband to an evaluation hospital, where dementia patients are treated. I was required to sign a promissory note stating that I would petition the superior court immediately for guardianship of my husband, or else they would release him from the hospital. Are you kidding me? The man has dementia. He does not even know my name and you are threatening to release him? I had to obtain separate attorneys to represent each of us, testify in court, and pay over $5,000 in attorney's fees in 1998.

Laws do vary from state to state, so do your homework, and check with an elder law attorney before your loved one's dementia progresses too far. Until my husband was in the last stage of dementia, almost every expense, except those provided by Medicare, was paid out-of-pocket.

If I had it to do over again, I would not have admitted my husband to this hospital. The staff was informative and supplied me with many statewide services and resources. They also drugged Red into a stupor and recommended immediate placement into a nursing home upon discharge. The poor guy was transformed overnight from a hyperactive child to a zombie. Thankfully, his geriatric psychiatrist was able to undo the damage by means of better drug management. Our geriatric psychiatrist prescribed a combination of medications to help control his horrendous behavioral issues while preserving his quality of life. Patience may be a virtue, but I had reached the bitter end. It took a couple of months to figure out which medications worked best, but ultimately, it was well worth the wait.

Creative investing and finances were my husband's forte during the first ten years of our marriage. Within ten seconds, this burden was dropped in my lap. Like the village idiot, I had allowed him to continue assuming financial responsibility even though I was aware something might be wrong. After all, he was the one with the MBA. Subsequent to his diagnosis, I discovered the financial mess we were in as a result of Red's illness and my denial. I decided the best thing for me to do, given I am not a financial wizard, was to transfer our existing bank accounts and income to one financial institution in order to consolidate our funds. Our trust attorney and professional financial advisor were willing to work with us to build a financial plan that fit our needs. Once this step was completed, I was on my way to feeling a lot more secure about our future.

Our first neurologists recommended signing up

with Safe Return and making or obtaining an identification card. I felt this was a bit premature, but I was wrong. My husband argued with anyone—including police officers. One time he snuck out on his bike when I was using the restroom and wound up at a pet store wanting some yard equipment fixed. After several similar incidents, I alerted my neighbors and local businesses within a five-mile radius to call our home when my husband arrived on their doorstep. You can't imagine how many calls I received the first three or four years after his diagnosis. We both carried his ID card in our wallets.

I will forever be hoarse due to the ear-splitting screaming my vocal cords endured until I sought help. As a dementia caregiver, I survived rage, broken ribs, decayed teeth, root canals, weight gain, depression, tendonitis, cortisone shots, and shoulder surgery. Caregiving is backbreaking. Is there a lesson here? It is survival of the fittest; ask for help.

Your journey will take more patience and courage than you have ever required in your life. It is the ultimate commitment. Hospice of the Valley advises to: "Anticipate, rather than react." Hope for the best, prepare for the worst.

Alzheimer's Association
24-hour helpline: 1-800-272-3900
Email address: info@alz.org

TAKE CARE OF YOURSELF

Remember how the flight attendant instructs you to put the oxygen mask on yourself before placing the mask on your child in case of an emergency? Bottom line, your loved one's survival depends on you.

After the initial preparation and chaos, slow down. Take it one day at a time. Do not overwhelm yourself with data and research until you are emotionally prepared. Take time to meet your needs as well as those of your loved one. Keep your home life uncomplicated and communication with your loved one simple. This means minimal, clear tasks, no multiple-choice questions, only questions that require a yes or no answer. Create and maintain a relaxed daily routine for both of you.

I encourage you to fill out the Caregiver Inventory Grief Form in *Appendix B* during the early stage of your caregiving journey. It is critical to assess your mental and emotional health by filling out this personal evaluation form before life gets out of control. Please share your results with your primary care physician.

"Adopt the pace of nature. Patience is her success."
—Ralph Waldo Emerson

LAUGHING

Virginia Pasquarelli

My loved one has dementia.
It's not easy to laugh.
Nothing seems funny
when my life's torn in half.

What's funny about silence
and losing the way?
I can hardly get out of bed
at the start of each day.

But sometimes I find it,
the ability to smile,
and it makes life bearable
for just a while.

He couldn't say "I love you"
but he still said "Damn."
He threw his tennis shoes
in the garbage can.

He became incontinent,
I became the Queen of Poop.
He forgot what a spoon was
and used a fork in his soup.

He came out of the bedroom
with shirt but no pants,
we had to do some hiding
because he tasted the plants.

Sometimes I laugh
and I don't even know why.
But I know if I didn't
all I would do is cry.

CHAPTER TWO

Behavioral Issues

Behavior problems emerge in the early stages of dementia and are frequently the most difficult and trying aspect of caregiving. In fact, having to deal with these issues is one of the leading causes of caregiver burnout. Dementia is in control and will prevail. Therefore, it is imperative you stay ahead of the disease and have a clear plan in place for managing difficult times. There will be difficult times. Recognize and accept change.

The following terminology is often used by physicians when evaluating and treating the behavior of a dementia patient:

- **Affect** is feeling or emotion evident by facial expression or body language.
- **Aphasia**, as defined in Webster's English Dictionary, is "a defect or loss of the power of

expression by speech, writing, or signs, or a defect or loss of the power of comprehension of spoken or written language."

- **Apraxia of speech** is caused by damaged parts of the brain related to speaking. The patient has trouble arranging and performing sounds in syllables and words.

- **Catastrophic reactions** are stress-related outbursts and a product of brain damage. The patient overreacts to circumstances beyond his or her control or comprehension.

- **Confabulations** occur when the patient fills the holes in his or her memory with fabrications he believes to be factual.

- **Delusion** is a perception thought to be true by the person experiencing it, although the perception is in reality wrong.

- **Dysphagia** is difficulty swallowing.

- **Emotional Lability (EL)** occurs when a patient exhibits rapid and drastic changes in his or her emotional state (such as laughing, crying, or anger) inappropriately and without a clear reason. It is defined as the inability to control one's expression of emotions.

- **Hallucinations** are a strong perception of an event or object when no such situation is present; hallucinations may occur in any of the senses.

- **Illusion** is a perception that occurs when a

sensory stimulus is present but is incorrectly perceived and misinterpreted, such as hearing the wind and believing someone is crying.

- **Insight** is defined as the ability to understand one's own problems.
- **Judgment** is the cognitive process of reaching a decision or drawing a conclusion.
- **Pica** is an eating disorder characterized by the repeated eating of non-nutritive substances over a period of one month or longer. Patients may eat non-edible objects such as paint, plaster, dirt, or laundry detergent.
- **Word salad (also called "disambiguation")** is a string of words that loosely resemble language, and may or may not be grammatically correct, but have no meaning.

There is a reason for a dementia patient's infuriating behavior. As the caregiver, your challenge is to determine the cause of the behavior, relax the patient, and diffuse the situation. Listed below are a few reasons for the patient's behavior:

- Agitation
- Anger
- Anxiety
- Boredom
- Constipation
- Depression

- Dirty diapers
- Distress
- Fatigue
- Fear
- Frustration
- Hunger or thirst
- Illness
- Medication side effects
- Noise
- Overstimulation
- Pain
- Showering

When our caregiver, Michelle, would try to help Red with his shower, he would grab the nozzle and spray her with water. After Michelle got soaked several times, we installed a cheap waterproof radio in his shower. We turned on the radio when he got in the shower and followed the music to the best of our ability. Who knows why he would spray Michelle with water? It could have been that he did not know what to do when he was in the shower, a fear of water, or that he liked to see Michelle react. In any case, the radio prevented him from doing it again, and this simple solution became a very useful tool in our house.

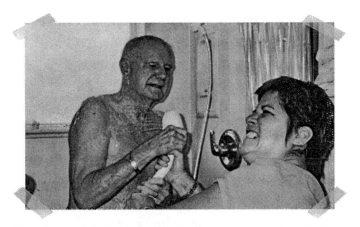

This is a photograph depicting anger and agitation, as Red (middle-stage) turns the shower nozzle on our caregiver, Michelle.

Every dementia patient's behavior is unique, yet comparable. You will have to experiment to determine what works best for you and your loved one when faced with behavior problems. Avoid confrontation and/or arguing. Below are many of the behavioral challenges Red and I dealt with, along with our attempts at solutions.

Agitation

You will find an agitation-rating questionnaire called the Cohen-Mansfield Agitation Inventory (CMAI) in *Appendix B*. The questionnaire consists of 29 questions in reference to your loved one's behavior. I suggest filling it out and sharing it with your physician. It will help the physician evaluate the patient so he or she can provide immediate treatment for current and impending behavioral problems.

Aggression

As we discussed earlier in this chapter, there are many reasons why dementia patients act aggressively. For example, they may be frustrated. They may want to leave a situation that they perceive as uncomfortable. They may be trying to communicate an idea, but cannot. They may also be acting aggressively because they feel despair, anguish, or agitation over their impossible situation. Undesirable behavior is often a result of a patient's inability to articulate his or her needs. Aggression and agitation may be exhibited through many behaviors: physical aggression, pacing, yelling, swearing, or whining, just to name a few.

Depending on where the patient is displaying the aggression, try using one or more of the following distraction techniques. Your loved one may require a calm environment, in which case some of these suggestions may result in unnecessary agitation. You must determine what will work in your unique situation.

Distraction Techniques

1.   Sing to your loved one; any song that comes to

mind in any type of voice that you can muster! A fun song to sing is the theme song to the 1965 CBS television show, *Green Acres*, written by Vic Mizzy. Sing loud, sing proud— unless it begins to agitate your loved one. No one is going to care what you sound like. It may help to distract and calm your loved one and relieve some of the stress you've both been experiencing. With any luck you will both end up laughing. Laughter is contagious.

2. Play music on the stereo and test the patient's tolerance levels as far as volume control. My spouse blew the speakers numerous times. Consider songs that will appeal to your loved one's generation. What kind of music did he or she listen to before becoming sick? Your loved one may not be able to talk, but he or she may still be able to sing. Consider Glen Miller, Nat King Cole, or Frank Sinatra. If the patient once loved musicals, why not put on *The Sound of Music*, *Phantom of the Opera*, or *South Pacific*. Music therapy was our best pacifier. Cirque du Soleil DVDs and Hamster Dance were house favorites.

3. Dance. Do you know any dance moves? It really doesn't matter because the purpose

of dancing is to distract your loved one. You can try dancing the jig, a little soft shoe, or the robot. Was either of you a cheerleader? You can try some cheers to sidetrack your loved one. The wilder and more animated, the better. Remember, the purpose of your dance or cheer is to distract the patient and redirect.

4. Offer your loved one a favorite food or some water. Offer snacks that might appeal to a toddler—soft and easy to chew—such as animal crackers, Cheerios, Fig Newtons, smoothies, chocolate, cereal bars, instant breakfasts, pudding, or peanut butter on crackers. Always consider the choking factor when choosing snacks. Stay away from nuts.

5. Take your loved one by the hand and go for a walk around the block, in the backyard, or even just down the hallway.

6. Make eye contact with your loved one, laugh with him or her, and give lots of hugs and kisses if he or she will tolerate human touch.

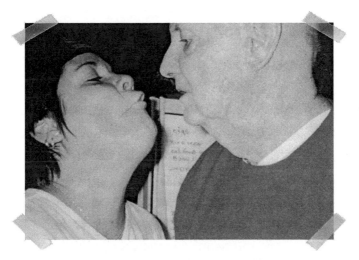

7. Offer your loved one a musical toy. The patient might try to eat toy parts, so purchase toys appropriate for a two-year-old.

8. Some studies report that aromatherapy has a significant effect on releasing agitation, with no side effects. The most commonly-used scents are lemon balm, to stimulate, and lavender oil, to calm. Be aware that anything that looks colorful or smells inviting may end up in the patient's mouth.

9. Give the patient a hand, foot, shoulder, or head massage. Warm the lotion slightly in the microwave. Do not set lotions within the patient's reach. He or she may drink it.

10. Take your loved one on a car ride around the neighborhood.

If your loved one is acting aggressively in public, where many of these options may not be immediately available, quietly take his or her hand and leave. Admittedly, this is easier said than done.

I rarely took my spouse out alone. During one trip to Home Depot, I sustained four broken ribs dragging my husband away from an intimidated, very pregnant check-out girl. In the beginning, I seemed to learn everything by mistake or injury. You really need backup in most cases if you are going to survive a trip to the store. My spouse touched and ate everything in the produce and candy sections, including shoplifting candy bars right in front of the cashier. I had some 'splaining to do, but had a good laugh in the end—well, maybe the next day.

Arguing as a Result of Presumed Dishonesty

Delusions, hallucinations, illusions, or confabulations may cause arguing as a result of your belief that your loved one is lying. Do not correct or challenge him or her. Agree and go do something else. Always take the easy way out unless it puts you or the patient in harm's way. Back off until the patient calms down.

Catastrophic Reactions

A catastrophic or overreaction may be caused by stress, fear, anger, frustration, or confusion, as well as by the patient's underlying illness and pain, or an onslaught of choices. Your loved one may react immediately by screaming, laughing, crying, or demonstrating aggressive behavior. The tendency to overreact is part of the disease. In my spouse's case, catastrophic reactions disappeared as the dementia progressed.

When catastrophic reactions occur, you calmly and promptly need to:

- Identify the behavior
- Resolve the situation before it worsens
- Make note of what triggered the behavior

Confabulations

Confabulations can be defined as the creation of false memories. These memories may have some truth woven in the story and they may not. In any case, the patient believes that what he or she is saying did truly happen. If your loved one begins to describe experiences that you know never took place, do not disagree with them and do not try to set them straight. You will never win. Just smile and nod your head. You do not need to correct or argue with the patient about what is true and what is not. It will just end with your feelings getting hurt, the patient getting angry, or worse, a catastrophic reaction. Pacify your loved one whenever possible. (I had no idea my husband was a clog dancer in his youth!)

Dressing the Patient

While the patient can still dress himself, let him do so. Allow the patient to remain independent for as long as it is feasible. It will give him or her a sense of pride and accomplishment and help avoid an unnecessary confrontation. As the disease progresses, your loved one may start wearing odd combinations of clothes. Who cares? Get over it! Let it go. Pick and choose your battles. It's not hurting anyone and no one is in danger. Laugh and take a picture for your photo album.

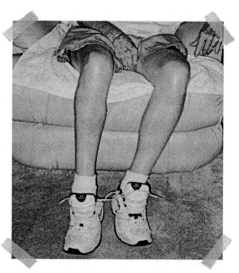

Middle-stage dressing can be a challenge, 2002

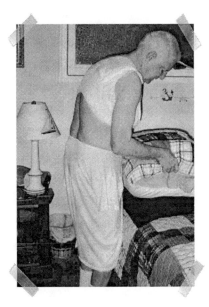

Late-stage dressing will be a challenge! 2005

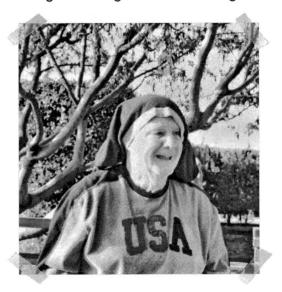

Eating, Food Obsessions, and Oral Fixation

There is a parallel between food, eating, and degeneration in the brain. Food may not smell or taste the same to the patient. The appetite control system may start to malfunction as cells deteriorate, resulting in distinct peculiar eating behaviors, overeating or not eating, and dehydration. As the condition progresses, your loved one must be supervised at every meal. Swallowing problems, along with pocketing and hoarding food, will increase the risk of malnutrition, choking, and aspiration (the inhalation of foods, beverages, saliva, or mucus into the lungs).

The first two to three years following the diagnosis, the only thing my husband would eat was Fry's fried chicken, bananas, and chocolate. His food likes and dislikes changed radically until I realized that he did not know the difference between something edible and a Styrofoam plate. He consumed cigarette butts, placemats, sea shells, dog barf, bar soap, dishwashing liquid, salad dressing, dog food, cat food, hair products, spray paint, liquid nails, trash, my checkbook registry—*anything!* We finally learned to have a plate full of snacks and water or juice next to his chair. We fed him many small meals consisting of finger foods, and focused primarily on hydration. Supply your loved one with water in order to maintain his or her fluid balance.

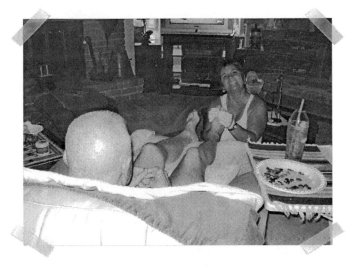

Note the snack tray and plastic glass with a straw. As time progressed, Red saturated his snack tray with water from Sippy cups. He became my sweet baby boy.

There is no specific diet for dementia, only proper nutrition. Red would touch, sniff, and taste everything within arm's reach. If the kitchen sink had fit into his mouth, he would have eaten it. Almost overnight his sense of smell was magically altered and enhanced. The scents he used to find repulsive were now irresistible. His caregiver, Michelle, witnessed him chasing me around a large tree in the backyard, index finger extended, insistent that I smell whatever foul odor was on the end of it. I knew what it was...that's why I ran.

As the dementia progressed, we focused on increasing Red's caloric intake versus achieving a balanced diet. Most dementia patients will begin to drop weight fast in the later stages of dementia. I say, let them have their chocolate, butter, and heavy cream.

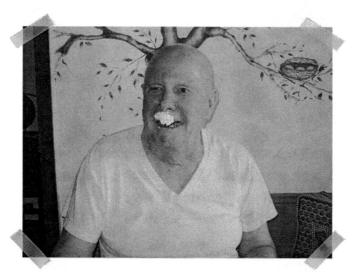

Eating with hands became the new normal.

Fixation

Dementia patients may focus on one issue they deem problematic. In our case, one of Red's many concerns was the trees in our front yard. He wanted them removed yesterday. It was the only thing he focused on for months. Next, it was his driver's license, and driving in general. He would not take no for an answer even though I explained that we (translation: I) were liable as his caregiver because I was aware he had a medical condition.

From experience I learned that, indeed, I was wasting my breath with numerous explanations. Red had no idea what I was talking about, nor did he care. It took me at least a year or two of drama to grasp that concept. Dementia patients are as self-absorbed and needy as a young child. It is not their fault, it's the dementia. You cannot change this behavior, you can only try to redirect or distract your loved one. The sooner you learn this lesson, the easier it is on the both of you.

Following the Caregiver

For several years, Red and I were attached at the waist. In hindsight, I believe this behavior was caused by feelings of insecurity and fear. Dementia can be very isolating for the patient and family alike.

Choose the path of least resistance to figure out the cause, distract and redirect the patient, and if all else fails, entice him to rest in his favorite chair with a snack.

Hoard and Hide

Yard art, jewelry, knickknacks, *everything*, is fair game for hoarding and hiding. When your head is turned, your loved one may abscond with your most precious pieces and hide them away, never to be found again.

It may be his or her attempt to regain control, or a result of mere boredom, confusion, fear, and isolation—regardless, it is *not* out of spite. Keep your eyes peeled for his or her favorite hiding places. Lock all medications, dangerous cleaning supplies, car keys, and anything you do not want to vanish into thin air away for safekeeping. If your loved one can still read, try signage around the house. You may want to designate a closet or drawer accessible to the patient as an area filled with all his or her favorite things.

When I asked Red where such and such was, he had no idea what I was talking about. To this day, objects I thought were lost forever still turn up. Red did not tolerate disorder or clutter.

Inappropriate Reactions

A normal reaction to a traumatic experience might be to cry, but the patient is laughing. When this happens the first time, your feelings will be hurt—especially if you're injured or up a tree as I was.

One morning, I was trimming a tree in the front yard when I noticed my husband laughing and trotting off to the shed with my ladder. Obviously, he did not like "clutter" in the yard. Even after a half an hour of screaming, Red didn't know what I was saying, nor did he care. Of course the whole neighborhood heard my earsplitting expletives. A neighbor took pity on me and retrieved the ladder so I could get down from the tree.

From that day forward, I only did yard work when Red was at daycare.

Judgment and Insight

Diminished judgment and insight impair decision-making, the patient's recognition of the consequences of inappropriate behavior as well as his or her safety, and the ability to focus and plan ahead.

Every dementia caregiver will accumulate his or her own list of amusing anecdotes, conundrums, and catastrophic experiences. Time and time again I learned the hard way due to my own errors in judgment. It is very difficult to take everything away from your loved one. Do not trust the judgment of a dementia patient with financial decisions, driving, handling sharp objects, cooking, or interacting with strangers.

A few anecdotes from my own experience:

- Strangers off the street were cordially invited into our home for a beer while I was at work.
  Solution: I quit my job.

- When my head was turned or I was in the bathroom, Red would disappear on foot or on his bicycle to Walgreens to beg complete strangers to give him their cars.

> **Solution:** I duct taped him to a chair—just kidding. The only thing I could do was hire a full-time caregiver and consider fencing in our home.

- A group of us witnessed Red trying to mow the lawn with our vacuum cleaner after I had given our lawn mower away.

  > **Solution**: I gave all dangerous gardening tools away and hid the vacuum cleaner.

- Red stalked and harassed our attorney. I sent flowers to our attorney to say I was sorry for the inconvenience and was still subjected to verbal abuse for not controlling my husband.

  > **Solution:** I switched attorneys.

- Red filled our dishwasher with dishwashing liquid, flooding the kitchen numerous times. Eventually this burnt up the dishwasher motor.

  > **Solution:** I bought a new, cheap dishwasher and hid the knob in a locked kitchen cabinet. Now why didn't I think of that with the first one?

- Due to limitless flushing, his toilet overflowed and flooded the laundry room.

  > **Solution:** I turned off the toilet valves.

- He broke every clock in our home by over-winding them.

    Solution: I removed and hid every clock in the house.

- The local clock shop was a favorite haunt of Red's. Clientele were scared away by his delight in public flatulence.

    Solution: I handed the shop employee my computer-generated card that read, "My husband has a brain disorder. Thank you for your patience." I coined this my "Yikes Card."

- 110 degree temperatures in Arizona did not stop my husband from jumping on his bicycle, briefcase in hand, and cycling 10 miles in 10 minutes to our financial advisor's office.

    Solution: I locked the bikes in our shed. When Red broke the shed locks to retrieve his bike, I donated the bikes to the Boys and Girls Club.

Each of these deeds was accomplished on the sly, or by outright lying to my husband. After a while, I was not sure who the demented one was. What had happened to my problem-solving instincts? Why hadn't I seen this coming? I had been convinced I was prepared for the worst.

This is the effect caregiving can have on you; your own sense of logic becomes strained. I can't believe I waited so long—too long—to ask for help. It was time to throw my pride out the window and get help.

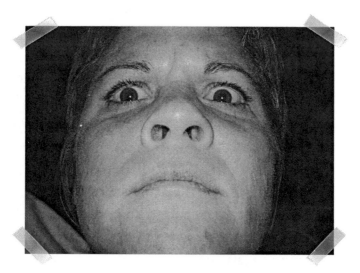

Our #1 caregiver, Michelle, is spent.

You will stumble on solutions if and when you are blessed with your own unique and challenging behavioral issues. Try, and I mean try, to measure your days in terms of accomplishments—not tribulations.

Medications

Every caregiver will have his or her own unique and challenging behavioral issues to deal with. Do not wait to take action until your own physical and mental health is affected. Consider working with a geriatric psychiatrist to find the appropriate medications for the patient, if necessary. Finding suitable medications can make a huge difference in the way a patient behaves. Medication will not cure the illness, but it can make the patient's behavior more manageable so your loved one is less of a threat to himself and others.

It will take time to find the right mix of medications for the patient to respond in a positive fashion. You need to be aware that some medications can have the opposite effect on dementia patients. As I mentioned previously, some doctors will prescribe Ativan (also known as Lorazepam) to treat anxiety and aggression. However, for dementia patients, this medication might produce the opposite effect; your loved one may become more agitated and hostile instead of calm.

A dementia patient must be monitored by the caregiver and physician for side effects produced by his or her medications. As a caregiver, stay well-informed. You may have to weigh your options and choose the lesser of two evils. I elected to medicate for my husband's safety and my sanity.

For up-to-date medication brochures, clinical trials, drug interactions, and drug assistant programs, refer to Appendix C.

Money

Red was adamant we close our bank accounts and hide our fortune in the top drawer of his dresser. Thankfully, I had already alerted our financial institution of my husband's illness with letters from his physician and financial power of attorney. *See Appendix B for a sample letter.*

In the good ole days, the Mister was very miserly. About four years after his diagnosis he took to rewarding strangers for their kindness with money and kisses. Personally, I believe this was his attempt at bribery.

As a solution, I removed the large bills from his wallet and replaced them with ten one-dollar bills. Red never knew the difference and could still bribe people with money and kisses.

Some enticing items my husband used to bribe our attorney in hopes of getting his driver's license reinstated were:

- One can of Sprite and one can of Pepsi
- A case of Hershey's candy bars
- Numerous photographs of random events in his life
- Paper towels
- One sleeve of Styrofoam cups
- Fifty dollars in cash

Nighttime

"Sun downing" is a term defined as an increase in agitation and behavioral issues in the late afternoon or evening. The progressive deterioration of the brain can also create challenging sleeping problems, such as:

- Apnea, or a pause in breathing while sleeping
- Disrupted sleep/wake timetables
- Nightmares
- Hallucinations
- Insomnia
- Movement of arms and legs
- Pacing
- Vocalization during sleep

Sleep disorders may be caused by a secondary disorder. Report any changes in behavior to the patient's physician. The following suggestions may help in the meantime.

- Establish a consistent evening sleep routine.
- Limit caffeine in the afternoon and evening.
- When exercise is possible, go for it.
- If feasible, regulate daytime napping until later stages of dementia.

In mid- to late-stage dementia we were able to get a hospital bed from hospice. We attached a baby fence to the end of the bed to keep Red from escaping in the middle of the night and wandering outside. Every door was alarmed and locked. Locks were placed above or below his reach. I elected to move into the guest bedroom so I could get some much-needed sleep, but kept an eye on him at night using a camera and baby television monitor. Most of the products mentioned are available at retailers, such as Target, for an affordable price.

Obsessive-Compulsive Disorder (OCD)

Obsessions, repetition, and compulsiveness are behaviors that make up this anxiety disorder, which can result from the progression of the dementia. OCD can take the form of verbal, behavioral, or motor repetitions. These compulsions may be deliberate, and can have a calming effect on dementia patients.

Due to short-term memory loss, a dementia patient may ask the same question over and over. His or her failing ability to cope causes anxiety and feelings of insecurity, making matters worse. The patient's anxiety will increase with your impatience. If possible, encourage your loved one to find the answer himself or herself. Leave the room and take five minutes for yourself when you can no longer contain your frustration.

As the dementia progressed, Red became mute. I really missed all those questions.

Parroting

Several years ago my husband walked into the middle of his daycare group. Instead of saying hi, he said the F-word in a deafening voice. Thankfully, the room erupted in laughter.

As Red's language skills diminished he would parrot me more, as a child learning to talk does. I learned I better watch what I say; he was still somewhat connected, and always listening. Funny thing, Red never uttered a swear word prior to dementia. I must have a real potty mouth when I'm angry.

Public Flatulence

What can I say? Hold your nose and laugh.

Sexually and Socially Uninhibited

Red loved to flash me or anyone else who would look. As a rule, this behavior was confined to the inside of our home since every door in our home was alarmed.

In January of 2006, Red's dream came true. He escaped unnoticed out the back door, naked as a jaybird. Our gardener chose not to embrace the vision of a naked, odiferous, 201-pound, seventy-two-year-old man. He just continued to blow the yard with his head down in embarrassment.

The only thing I could think to do was apologize and hand our gardener one of my "Yikes" cards. You will get your point across without embarrassing your loved one.

The "Yikes" card also applies to verbal and social missteps. My spouse's indiscreet comments to friends and family included:

- "These cookies taste awful. They're too hard!"
- "Are you leaving soon?"
- "Is this your stuff? Can I put it in your car now?"
- "I don't want to do this stuff."
- "Move, so I can put this in the dishwasher."

Spatial and Motor Skills

Dementia progression may result in a loss of spatial skills and visual perception. The brain's ability to interpret what the eyes see is impaired. Familiar tasks, such as pushing a grocery cart, sitting, dressing, cooking, cleaning, and eating independently may no longer be possible.

The patient may also lose facial and environmental recognition. My spouse spent hours looking in the mirror at himself, making faces. I honestly don't think he recognized his own image. Research confirms my theory. Dementia patients may not recognize their own reflections. As a result, they may feel threatened by or frightened of the person looking back at them. Try covering mirrors to avoid unnecessary distress and anxiety.

Red did not recognize family members for at least five years before he passed and was not capable of discriminating between men and women. Whoever was sitting in my favorite chair was his wife. Of course, initially I was hurt, until I realized that any warm body in my chair was his security blanket and a hand to hold.

Spitting

Always carry tissues or wet wipes—chances are, you'll need them.

Suspicion/Jealousy

Dementia patients may become suspicious or jealous of anyone and everyone. They may become concerned that other people are taking advantage of them or are out to hurt them in some way. The dementia patient might blame someone of stealing from him or her, when in fact the patient simply misplaced the item. To a large degree, this occurs due to failing memory combined with your loved one's decreased ability to recognize people.

Before rejecting your loved one's fears, make sure there is no validity to his or her claim. Avoid arguing and calmly comfort or distract the patient as best you can. Explain to others that any finger-pointing is a result of the dementia—friends, family, and strangers should not take these accusations personally.

For Red, any conversation I had with a male, in-person or on the phone, resulted in unyielding suspicions and jealous accusations. A short chat with the mailman would result in Red asking me countless questions, usually ending with, "Do you want to marry him?" This behavior, too, passed by the middle stage of dementia.

Urinating in Public

Like a lone wolf, my husband marked his territory from the Pacific Ocean to the Southwest desert, as well as every sink in our home, and several flower pots. To this day, I don't know what I could have done to prevent this behavior other than never take him anywhere.

Red's geriatric psychiatrist suggested we train his bladder by taking him to the bathroom every two hours. I thought it was a very good idea, but not too realistic. The best I could do was be prepared and observant.

I put together an emergency car kit that included the following items:

- Urinal/bed pan
- Disposable waterproof pads
- Change of clothes
- Wet wipes
- Diapers
- Garbage bags

Refer to Appendix B for a copy of my emergency car kit.

Urinating in Atypical Places

From 2001 until he was incontinent, Red urinated in the bathroom sink. All three bathroom sinks, never the toilets. I even had a higher sink installed in his bathroom, but to no avail. The only solution was to limit the mess he made by locking two of the bathrooms so he could not use them. For the remaining bathroom, I also put the lock on the outside of the door so he wouldn't lock himself in. Eventually, I removed the bathroom door altogether. It was not worth it to reprimand him or try and control this behavior. I kept a box of Clorox wipes on his sink for the occasion. He probably tried to eat them when I wasn't looking.

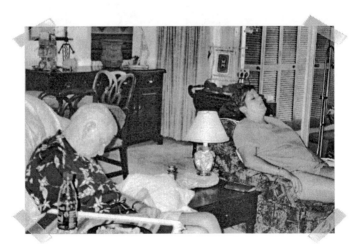

What a day!

My spouse's problematic behavior was challenging and unpredictable to say the least. Our struggles began years prior to the initial diagnosis and continued through the middle stages of dementia. Red was his own worst enemy, a danger to himself and others.

Often, finding a solution to behavioral problems happens through trial and error. Every dementia patient is different, but all share numerous similarities. It is normal to get frustrated, impatient, angry, even livid. If the day's events start to get to you, step back, and if possible, take a ten-minute timeout.

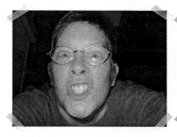 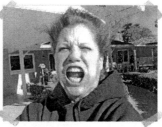

The author and #1 caregiver, Michelle, in 2005

A word to the wise: Put your glasses on *before* kissing a dementia patient, or you may come in contact with a booger or worse. (Again, the hard way...)

Take Care of Yourself

Maintain relationships with family and friends who have supportive, uplifting, and positive attitudes. Your family and friends can help you through your darkest days, so stay connected as much as possible. Reach out to someone at least once a week by writing a letter or email to keep up your friendships. Make sure your family and friends are aware you are eager to chat and ready to accept help.

Expect and accept the fact that you will lose the emotional support of at least some friends and family. Many people are intimidated, scared, or feel vulnerable because your situation could happen to them, either as a dementia patient or caregiver.

AARP Foundation Programs offers an excellent "Planning Guide for Families," available here:

http://assets.aarp.org/www.aarp.org_/articles/foundation/aa66r2_care.pdf.

To obtain a physical copy, call or write AARP Foundation Programs.
- Call: 1-888-687-2277, Monday through Friday, 7:00 a.m.–midnight EST
- Write: AARP, 601 E Street NW, Washington, DC 20049

TRYING

Virginia Pasquarelli

The one I love.
Losing words, losing
whereabouts, losing memories.
Not the same. What's wrong?

An exam room, a doctor.
Questions and answers.
So many fears.

Dementia.
Horrible word.
Our future, detonated.
What will happen?

Words are lost, whereabouts,
Memories gone.
He loses himself.

I am lost, too.
So much to do.
All by myself.
I try.

I try.
I learn this caring.
But I always knew
how to love.

Just a different
way to love now.
Diapers. Dressing.
Taxes. I try.

Each day
we get through
is one more day
we are together.

Dementia.
Horrible word.
But the love
is beautiful.

CHAPTER THREE

Managing Daily Living

According to the Alzheimer's Association, nearly fifteen million Americans, primarily family members, provide unpaid care for individuals with dementia. As a caregiver, you may feel ignored and unappreciated, but you are not alone. The goal of this chapter is to remind you that you cannot properly care for your loved one without help. That first call is the most difficult. Go ahead and make it.

The last two years of Red's life, I employed one full-time and one part-time caregiver. The three of us teamed up with hospice and provided all of my husband's basic needs around the clock. The following suggestions and recommendations worked for us, but may not be suitable for all dementia patients and caregivers. Every caregiver should evaluate the following information along with his or her physician to make informed choices that fit the patient's and caregiver's special needs.

The ability to perform Activities of Daily Living (ADL) is an essential part of measuring the competence of a person with dementia and is important in determining the diagnosis and assessing the disease's progression. In addition to diagnosis, the measurement of ADL performance allows for the evaluation of treatment effects, caregiver burden, and helps assess the need for caregiver intervention and assistance.

Activities of Daily Living

A typical list of Activities of Daily Living includes:

- Getting Dressed/Selecting Clothes
- Eating/Drinking
- Managing Finances
- Preparing Meals
- Maintaining an Interest In Hobbies
- Accomplishing Housework/Shopping
- Being Familiar with Spatial Orientation
- Taking Care of Personal Hygiene
- Retaining Speech/Comprehension
- Being Mobile
- Driving Skills
- Ability to Answer and Comprehend Telephone Calls

There are numerous methods used to measure the progression of dementia. Two of my preferred methods, Functional Assessment Staging (FAST) and The Clinical Dementia Rating (CDR), are scales available for your use in *Appendix B*. Please share the results with your physicians.

The following list of everyday activities will give you a sense of the most likely difficulties you will face as a caregiver, along with solutions based on my own experience with Red.

Bathing/Hygiene
Bathing

Bathing can be as traumatic for the caregiver as for the patient and has the potential to provoke a catastrophic reaction or aggressive behavior. Put yourself in your loved one's position. I personally would not enjoy being undressed and bathed by a stranger. I would be mortified. Until a structured routine is established, disruptive behavior is not an unusual response.

Remember to choose your battles. It might not hurt to put off a bath or shower for a day. Unfortunately, I have a bionic sense of smell. I could smell "it" even if he thought about "it." On occasion, I was known to spray my husband with Febreze until he was at last receptive to a bath.

Suggestions for Bath Time

- Be patient, flexible, sensitive, and gentle at all times.

- I recommend using a liquid soap for sensitive skin or a head-to-toe body wash.

- If your loved one is incontinent, I advise washing his or her bum using disposable wipes. It will save you from additional laundry or trips to the store to replace soiled wash rags. In the later stages, consider a no-rinse body wash.

- Organize and position everything you need for bathing within arm's reach: diapers, clean cloths, soap, shampoo, ointments, wet wipes, and a towel.

- Establish a regular bathing routine (time, day, type of bath).

- Encourage the patient to bathe himself or herself whenever possible. Of course, you must stay in the bathroom with the patient at all times.

- Use creative distraction techniques to make the patient comfortable. Music may sooth the savage beast—how about a sing-a-long?

- Be observant. Baths are an opportunity to check for bruising, skin irritations, rashes, infections—anything out of the norm.

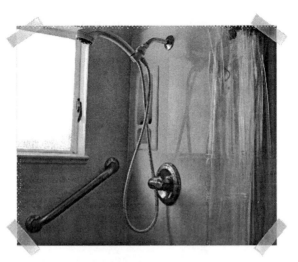

I recommend installing a flow control handheld shower attachment with an extra long hose and grab bars on two sides of the shower stall for additional support.

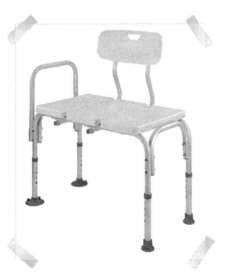

A transfer bench with a seat extension allows users to easily slide into the tub area.

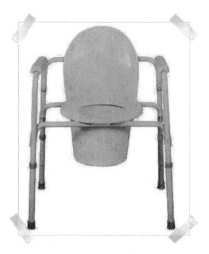

A 3-in-1 commode adjusts to different heights and may also be used in the shower once the pail is removed.

For safety, put a washable non-skid area rug on the floor next to the shower or tub. Have a spare trashcan or pail available in case of accidents. My husband inevitably had to potty the minute he was all cleaned up. We threw out a lot of rugs.

Brushing Teeth

I recommend gel toothpaste made with tea tree oil, which is excellent for gum health. If the patient is inclined to swallow the toothpaste, use a brand made for children to avoid any side effects such as nausea, vomiting, or diarrhea.

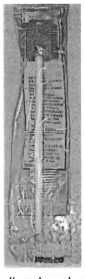

Toothettes are a disposable, ready-to-use foam brush, especially useful for removing debris.

The most efficient option is to use a child's electric or battery-run toothbrush. Do not stick your fingers in between the patient's teeth. I learned the hard way...ouch! In the later stage of dementia, Red would bite anything that found its way into his mouth. If you notice your loved one's gums are red, discolored, or bleeding, try the suggestions below.

- Colgate Peroxyl is an antiseptic oral cleanser that promotes the healing of oral irritations.
- Gly-Oxide is a leave-on antiseptic oral cleanser. Both Gly-Oxide and Colgate Peroxyl can be applied using Toothettes.
- A water pik will help dislodge leftover food debris.

Shaving

After Red's daily shaves resulted in numerous facial cuts, it was visibly time to add my husband's shaving to my own list of duties. Rather than take him to the barbershop and risk public agitation, I chose to set up a stress-free salon at home. To tackle the excess hair, I needed a couple of useful cutting tools, and most importantly, an electric razor. I chose to have fun with this daily chore. For several months we experimented with a mustache and goatee. His beauty makeover, of course, was very impractical. I had no idea what would get caught up in the additional facial hair.

Washing Hair

Most people like having their hair washed. However, many dementia patients fear having their heads covered with water. Listed below are a few options to make this chore easier on the caregiver and patient:

- Bathe and wash hair separately. On days when the patient only has to bathe, use a shower cap.
- Try a dry shampoo.
- Shampoo in the kitchen sink using a spray attachment.
- Use a hand-held shower attachment.
- Find a hairdresser who will come to the house.

Be aware that some medication can make hair oily or stinky, and can cause hair loss as well. We chose to give my husband a military cut using battery-operated shears. Just for fun, we even tried to dye it red, his natural color. Remember, a short haircut is much easier to keep clean.

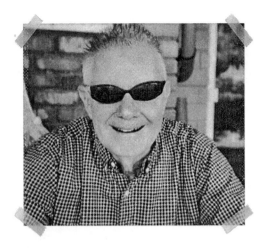

Cold Remedies

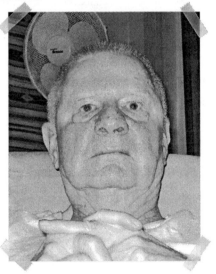

Breathe Right Strips worked a miracle on Red's stuffy nose, although they did give his nostrils the appearance of an ox. Goodie, a chance to laugh!

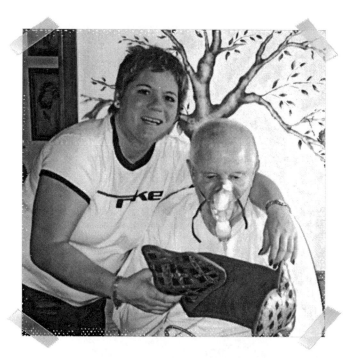

In his last year, Red would frequently get congested due to lack of mobility. Hospice provided us with a nebulizer and Lidocaine to help dry up his lungs and control his cough. Michelle secured his wandering hands with oven mitts to prevent him from disrupting the process.

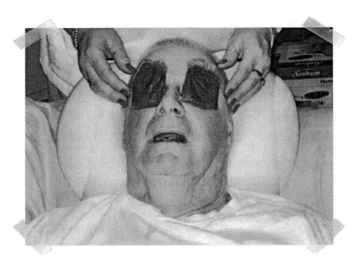

We applied cold damp tea bags on his eyes to reduce puffiness and sinus pressure. Who knows why, but he loved it.

Be sure to check with your loved one's geriatric psychiatrist or primary care doctor before using any over-the-counter medications. Sudafed and Afrin may increase confusion in dementia patients and trigger other adverse side effects as well.

Daycare

Adult daycare centers can be public, private, non-profit, or for-profit. The objective of a daycare center is:

- to provide dementia patients with the opportunity to get relief from the structure of home life, and receive mental, physical, and social stimulation.

- to give caregivers a much-needed break.

My husband's adult daycare center divided the patients into groups according to individual mental competency. They also provided caregivers with a monthly calendar. A typical calendar included:

- o A month's worth of daily menus
- o Mental stimulation games
- o Daily arts and crafts
- o Musical entertainment and sing-a-longs
- o Exercise
- o Birthday and holiday celebrations
- o Outings

My exhaustion and increasing lack of patience led me to seek out an adult daycare facility. I also felt that Red needed more stimulation than I was able to provide at home. Red's first day of daycare was a real guilt trip for me. The van arrived at 7:00 a.m. with one other poor soul riding shotgun. I felt so sorry for Red. I could tell he wasn't looking forward to the next few hours. I called the center a half hour later to let them know he had been fretting about the day.

Poor thing arrived home at 3:00 p.m. The whole experience had been very distressing for him. His initial reaction was, "I don't ever want to go there again! No one says anything, half of the people don't talk American, and nobody would talk to me."

"Do you have a headache?" I asked him. He didn't.

"Do you feel bad for the people at the center?" He admitted he did.

For the next hour, the drama queen faked fainting by running into door jambs and the refrigerator. By early evening, he said he felt better and agreed to visit the center again, if I went too.

Most facilities require a doctor's exam, TB test, and chest X-ray prior to allowing the patients to attend daycare. Every state has different licensing and patients' requirements.

Below is an example of the mental and physical competency list I made for my husbands daycare facility. You will want to create your own. I also included a photo of my husband for the facility to use as a reference.

Patient: Harold M. Scarff, aka "Red"
- Cognitive age: 12 to 18 months
- Late-stage frontotemporal dementia
- Inability to speak and comprehend
- Very stubborn
- Occasionally able to problem-solve
- Completely incontinent

Causes of Agitation:

- Boredom
- Soiled underwear
- A need to poop
- Hunger
- Thirst (he dehydrates easily)
- Exhaustion
- Pain

To Distract/Redirect:

- Play music (he likes it loud)
- Sing to him
- Dance with him
- Provide snacks or water
- Take him by the hand and walk
- Laugh while making eye contact
- Give him a musical toy

Requires:

- Total direction
- Supervised meals (cut food, preferably finger foods, into small pieces)
- A tablespoon for eating
- Provide him with his beverage after his meals or he will dump the liquid into his meal

Suggestions and Recommendations:

- Enlist the help of two people when changing his diapers.
- Do not put anything within arm's reach because Red will eat it.

- Do not put your fingers in Red's mouth. Use an implement, such as a tongue depressor.
- Do not use an oral thermometer because he will bite it.
- Eye contact, laughter, and human touch work well with Red. He does not like to be alone.
- Anything you might do to amuse a baby will likely work with Red.
- Red has NO fear; therefore he is a danger to himself as well as others.

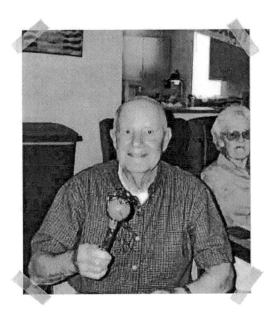

It's karaoke day at the daycare center.

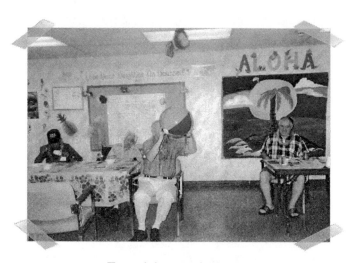

Exercising at daycare.

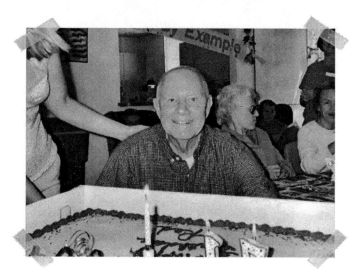

Happy Birthday, Redski.

As you're investigating adult daycare centers, make sure the facility is secure and can provide for a dementia patient. Call ahead and schedule a visit. Personally, I like the drop-in approach so the facility doesn't have time to clean up for my visit. A few items to consider once you're there:

- Days and hours of operation
- Eligibility requirements: Can they accommodate incontinent dementia patients?
- Patient age range
- Cost per day
- Any discounts, such as those for low-income clients
- Staff-to-patient ratio
- A typical month's worth of activities
- Number of years in business

If your loved one is incontinent, he or she needs to be changed, or at least checked, every two hours. Do not allow the daycare center to send your loved one home in dirty diapers or clothes. We sent a change of clothing and numbered diapers along with Red to make sure the daycare center staff were changing him. Ideally, the daycare center will have a washer, dryer, and showers available.

Some facilities may currently have too many clients, in which case they cannot give each individual the attention he or she needs. Be proactive and do your homework. You do not want your loved one to get sick (or unnecessarily discouraged) as a result of unsafe or unsanitary conditions.

Refer to Appendix B for an Adult Daycare Checklist.

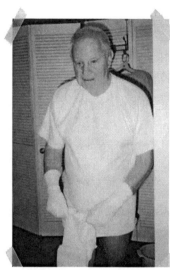

September 2005:
What a difference
four years made

Dressing Your Loved One

Hopefully by now you will be able to find humor in challenges such as this. For at least two years, my husband would not accept any help getting dressed. I tolerated this behavior and moved on to more important issues. I did draw the line when Red put his underwear on over his pants if we were venturing out. When he thought he did not have enough clothing in his side of the closet, he helped himself to mine. You should have seen him in high water parachute pants. In the late stage of dementia, we dressed him in pajamas and sweats. They were much easier to get off when it was time to wash the clothes or change the diapers, and these items were affordable as well.

Dressing an Incontinent Patient

To help a dementia patient stay as independent as possible, invest in easy-on, easy-off clothing. As time goes by, you will not only need to pick out your loved one's clothes, but you will also need to physically help him or her dress. Pull-on, stretchable, elastic-waist clothing such as sweatpants are great for those with dementia. I recommend pullover shirts, dresses, and skirts versus items with buttons or zippers. Other practical clothing suggestions include:

- Men's long brief underwear (excellent for keeping diapers and their contents in place)
- Skid-proof socks
- Slippers, slacks, or nightgowns with Velcro fasteners

Similar items may be purchased at online retailers such as Silverts.com. Silvert's Disabled Disability Clothing carries a full line of men and women's adaptive clothing.

A link and toll-free phone number are available in Appendix C under clothing resources.

Driving

Driving around town was one of my husband's favorite pastimes, so I had to have a game plan if I hoped to survive. I put together a car tool kit with everything I could possibly need for the worst-case scenario. I always carried a urinal with a lid on it so Red could relieve himself "on the spot."

You can find a copy of my car tool kit in Appendix B.

As my husband's dementia progressed, I could not take him in the car without a second caregiver in the passenger seat to supervise Red in the back-seat. He would grab the steering wheel or try to open the door. Activating the car door childproof locks and dead bolting his seat belt did not guarantee he would not unlock it. I secured his door and window hoping we would make it from point A to point B without a problem. Even then, he would reach over the seat to grab whatever he could.

Emergency Room Kit

As described in Chapter 1, a personal emergency room kit is essential for unexpected hospital or doctor visits.

For our kit, I made several copies of my spouse's medical insurance cards. I kept one in my wallet and one in his wallet for emergencies. The patient's Social Security number is usually on the Medicare card. In addition, I produced all of my records in large print so I could read them without my glasses. Trust me, you can never find your spectacles when you need them.

Always carry a letter from the patient's primary care physician stating that your loved one is under a doctor's care. Keep a copy of the letter in your emergency kit. You might also want to drop off a copy of this letter to your banking institution for their records; this will prevent your loved one from making an unanticipated financial decision.

Refer to Appendix B for a sample emergency room kit; an example of an advisory physician's letter can be found in Appendix B.

Exercise

Luck was with me when I found a trainer at the YMCA who was willing, for a price, to work with Red and supervise him while I completed my own routine. At this point in his progression my husband was almost mute, with about 5% comprehension, but he was still physically ready, willing, and able to exercise. With a prescription from his primary care physician I was able to write off the gym membership and his trainer.

In 2003, we completed the one-mile Alzheimer's Memory Walk. I think he thought I was going to ditch him because he insisted on holding hands. What a lovely bonus.

If your loved one is no longer able to walk, take him or her out in a wheelchair or transporter. For entertainment, I added a squeezable horn to the transporter for Red to use on daily walks around the block. Red loved the noise, and the motion itself exercised his hands.

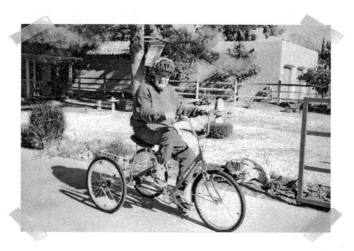

Christmas 2004. The problem with this scenario is that he did not know how to stop the bike. We got more exercise running beside his new bike braking for him!

Food and Hydration

In the early stage of dementia, expect food obsessions. My husband devoured fried chicken, candy bars, gum, and chocolate for a couple of years.

Choking, pocketing (storing food in one's mouth without swallowing), and dysphagia (difficulty swallowing) will become challenges. Do not force your loved one to eat. This can lead to aspiration (entry of food into the wind pipe), or worse. At times, the patient may even forget to eat. These issues are unpredictable.

Dementia eventually sets its own schedule. Don't fight it. Food tastes may change, and food obsessions may appear. Allow and encourage your loved one to retain his or her independence by feeding himself or herself. If your loved one is no longer able to use silverware, prepare finger foods, or cut his or her food into small pieces that the patient can pick up with his or her hands. Fixing a variety of finger food also has the advantage of giving you a clear idea of what currently appeals to the patient. Snacks in between meals will help improve food intake as well.

Do not rush meal time. Allow your loved one to eat at his or her own pace, focus on foods that minimize the risk of choking, and supervise all meals.

Easy Snack Ideas
- Bite-size crackers
- Fruit (dried or fresh)
- Soft cereal bars
- Dry cereal
- Smoothies
- Ensure
- Boneless chicken strips

Red and I learned to keep life simple and take it one day at a time. I found uneaten food hidden in boxes of trash bags, my purse, wherever. Flexibility is a must because you have no idea what to expect next. In the past, I had been an anal, nitpicking perfectionist. Dementia changed that, and I'm glad. Life is too short.

My husband put on at least twenty to thirty pounds through the middle stage of his illness. I regarded it as emergency flab we may need in the near future, and it turns out we did.

Facial/Object Recognition

Dementia patients share a deficit in their ability to recognize facial expressions, as well as familiar people, places, and objects. This deficiency can terrify a loved one (and no doubt the caregiver, as well).

By 2001, my husband no longer recognized people who were not in his life on a daily basis, including family members. I purchased a blank picture book and included labeled photographs of relatives and close friends. We spent time looking at these, as well as creating scrapbooks that attempted to preserve any of Red's remaining memories. I can't say it helped much other than to pacify me. Over time, I learned to live with being called "Honey, Honey," "Hey, lady," and, "Mom." He had long forgotten my name.

Fevers

If the patient's brain ceases to regulate body temperature, the caregiver may need to reduce a fever for the patient.

Hospice recommended liquid Tylenol every four hours as a prophylactic measure for fever or pain. We also applied moist, cool towels to pressure points in the neck and wrist. Liquid Tylenol made a tremendous difference in my husband's quality of life, especially in the late stage of dementia.

A sudden high fever can also produce fever blisters (also known as cold sores). Ask your pharmacist or physician to recommend a product to treat fever blisters. The proper medication will ensure a shortened healing time.

Financial Institutions

Even though I was prepared from the get-go, I still ran into problems with the bank. Financial institutions will require the proper paperwork to be on file, including your current financial power of attorney. In one instance, they insisted I bring my spouse to the bank for his signature. Mind you, they had a power of attorney (POA) on file and a letter from his primary care doctor. I reiterated that he was mute, did not know his name, and was not capable of providing his signature. I ended up having to bring him to the bank, and with his hand in mine, we wrote a large X for his signature. I could tell he was humiliated, and I was furious. The bank manager then proceeded with his best sales pitch: "You need to get a conservatorship for your husband, and we can help you set that up." That same day I transferred our funds to a different financial institution and lodged a severe complaint.

Don't let anyone take advantage of you or your loved one. During this time, you are both at your most vulnerable. Do not cave in only because it makes your life easier. Beware of financial institutions, caregiving agencies and personnel, home repairmen, or anyone who offers you a service you don't need, want, or cannot afford.

Holidays and Travel

Dementia patients often enjoy day trips to a favorite place. My husband loved short rides as long as we returned to the ole homestead by dusk. I attempted several overnight trips that ended in the emergency room. I was stubborn or in denial, learning the hard way, as usual.

Overnight vacations quickly became a thing of the past. The patient's stress, agitation, and confusion, combined with the caregiver's planning, packing, and exhaustion, makes the whole experience a nightmare. Bottom line, a dementia patient is much more comfortable in familiar surroundings, and you will be too.

Holidays have the additional disadvantage of disrupting a dementia patient's routine, which can lead to a change in behavior. Eventually, I decided to celebrate Christmas in our home rather than go through long-distance travel. Even adding a new decoration to our usual décor caused a catastrophic reaction. If it does not put anyone in harm's way, most things are not worth the fight.

Home Aides

Home care providers allow a patient to stay in his or her home longer. Aides offer a variety of services, such as providing the patient with supervision, personal care, activities, exercise, and medical needs, and may also help with the housekeeping, shopping, and cooking. Home care can be a lot less expensive than a nursing home or an assisted-living facility, especially for caregivers who need only a couple hours of help a day.

The most expensive option is to hire an employee from a home-health agency. The agency will take care of the aide's withholding taxes and provide benefits. They will find a substitute on days your aide cannot come. The agency may also provide the aide with insurance and arrange for ongoing training. A certified aide who is an agency employee will cost somewhere from $17 to $25 an hour. The more trained the aide, the costlier he or she will be.

Reliable agencies will conduct an in-home interview and assess your loved one's needs. Do your research. Most health care agencies are businesses rather than non-profit organizations as many of them lead you to believe. Services, training, and fees vary among caregivers and agencies. I was able to negotiate a reduced rate with an agency by signing a one-year contract.

You will also save money by hiring an aide on your own. You might find one through the newspaper, an online service, a friend, or your church. I found word-of-mouth (from those I trusted) the best way to go. Expect to pay from $10 to $18 an hour. If you go this route, you will be an employer. As a result, you may need to obtain a Federal ID number and submit a quarterly unemployment tax and wage report. Typically, Medicare doesn't pay for home care, but you can use it as a health care tax write-off.

If you do hire an aide on your own, meet with the potential aide in your home first. Be prepared with a list of questions. It's a good idea to have another person present so that the two of you can discuss the interview afterward. Two heads are better than one. Get references, call them, and do a background check. You are entrusting your loved one's life and your own well-being with this individual. You don't want to end up with more problems than you already have. Once you hire your aide, prepare a daily schedule of duties along with a checklist, so your expectations for the caregiver are always clear.

For more home aide and caregiving resources, see Appendix C.

Incontinence

When there is a decline in memory as a result of dementia, incontinence will eventually be an issue. By this point, if you have not already sought help and developed a sense of humor, now is the time! In many cases, this is the straw that breaks the camel's back.

Incontinence may be caused by a medical problem, a urinary tract infection, or prostate enlargement. The patient should be assessed by a physician to rule out any underlying medical problems, and I encourage you to keep a record of anything unusual for the doctor to review as part of the process.

Your loved one may not recognize the bathroom or might forget how to use a toilet, so be patient. There will be mishaps, confusion, disgust, humiliation, embarrassment, and even chaos, especially in the initial onset of incontinence. Get help to manage this problem and take many time-outs for yourself.

I learned a few tricks through the years to prevent disasters related to incontinence. I was known in my social circle as the Queen of the Poop-O-Rama.

- As mentioned previously, we turned off the valves behind the toilet so he could have only one flush. This was a simple yet effective solution.
- All but one bathroom were kept locked to localize the mess.
- We removed my husband's bathroom door to prevent him from locking himself in. This also allowed us to better monitor his need for help.
- Prior to using diapers, we numbered the toilet paper squares to see if Red was actually cleaning his bottom after every bowel movement. As I suspected, he was not. At this moment, his privacy came to an abrupt halt.

One of my online group members experimented with diet and stool softeners. He actually got his wife's bowel movements timed to between 2:00 and 3:00 p.m. every day. I was inspired, but in the end, this potential solution did not work with my husband.

Some dementia patients will take to playing with their excrement. By this point, your loved one is incontinent and needs to be monitored closely. Experiment with creative dressing to prevent this behavior. We dressed Red in a couple layers of clothing on the bottom half. It kept the excrement in the diaper and he was too lazy to take the extra clothing off.

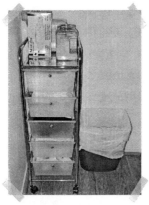 This is a photo of our price-less rolling bath and incon-tinence storage unit. It con-tained everything we could possibly need to change and bathe my husband: T-shirts, extra wipes, dia-pers, diaper pads, oint-ments, anti-skid socks, and disposable gloves. I purchased this item at Target. It saved us time, energy, and patience. We also stored disposable gloves in a wide-mouth plastic jar for easy access.

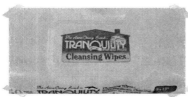 I highly recommend Tranquility Cleans-ing Wipes for adults. Hospice will provide their own wipes, but they are not near the quality or size, and do not have the absorption potential.

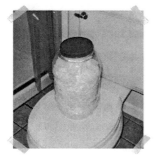 We saved a two-gallon clear cookie jar for cleansing wipes. They are too difficult to manage in an emergency while still in the package. One cleansing wipe never does the job!

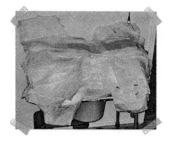

We layered and stacked a dozen diapers and liners so we were ready to go at a moment's notice.

Protective ointment helps treat and prevent rashes associated with diaper use or continued exposure to feces, urine, or both. It also helps seal out wetness. We experimented with a variety of over-the-counter baby care products that proved very effective. Your physician or hospice care nurse will be able to provide you with products or product recommendations for adult care incontinence use.

For maximum protection, I recommend "Tranquility All Through the Night" disposable diapers with side tabs. They are much easier to put on and take off the patient. The pull-up brief is sufficient while the patient is still somewhat cognizant. In addition, I lined the inside of his diaper with a "Tranquility Pad" as an extra leakage safeguard.

Finding a product to eliminate unpleasant odors is a must. Purchase a product that kills 99.99% of germs. I used a concentrated product called Odoban that cleaned, disinfected, and deodorized every corner of our home, including drains. This product is not to be used on skin or patients' clothing. To find a safe and reliable product, get a recommendation from the local hospital, nursing home, or adult daycare centers.

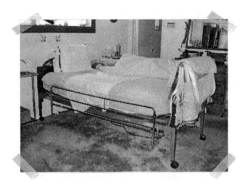

Bed

You may want to purchase tuck-in, waterproof, mattress pads. Washable pads are available for almost any bed size and do not move around under the patient. We kept clean, spare pads at the foot of the bed for convenience and emergencies. It is more cost-effective to buy the washable pads since the disposable pads do not hold much liquid. Make sure you get more than one so you can swap them out during a wash. I used the waterproof overlays on Red's chair and in the car as well.

We kept a large trashcan in the bedroom and changing area lined with at least six to eight trashcan liners in each. It makes for fast and easy disposal whether you fling it out the back door or patiently deposit it in the dumpster.

As for disposable diapers, they come in a variety of sizes. In the initial stage of incontinence, we used the pull-up briefs. As the dementia progressed, we switched to a heavy-duty refastenable tab diaper. They were much easier to check and change. Hospice provides anything you need, but be warned: in our case, their diapers did not accommodate a bladder the size of an elephant. I bought a pair of adult rubber panties to put on over Red's diapers. I do not recommend it. Within 24 hours, I had created an inflamed red rash around his legs and waist. Just one more learning experience...

Change an adult's diaper as soon as you notice it is soiled to help prevent skin rashes and to make your loved one more comfortable. It is wise to check his or her diaper a minimum of every two hours. Wash, dry well, and treat any rash immediately.

Prior to total incontinence, there will be mishaps. The timing and locale may be a mystery. The possibilities are endless, so stay vigilant.

For more incontinence resources, see Appendix C.

Mail

Red would often collect the mail and dump it in our neighbor's trashcan. I was forced to buy a lockable mailbox and mount it on a fence post. To keep him pacified and feeling productive, I purchased a fake mailbox and stationed it inside our gate, filling it with throwaway catalogs and junk mail. As I have mentioned before, dementia patients can be obsessive about many things. You must be aware of where your loved one is at all times.

Medications

Currently, there is no cure for dementia, only medications to treat behavioral changes such as agitation and depression. A small group of approved drugs may temporarily improve some symptoms and slow the progression of the disease. One of the downsides can be the unwanted side effects, such as drooling, hair loss, oily hair, and skin rashes. Patient benefits versus side effects must be discussed with your loved one's physician. Weekly or monthly monitoring should be a part of your patient care routine. I am a firm believer in using medication to improve a patient's quality of life rather than to sedate him or her, unless absolutely necessary.

Steer clear of over-the-counter sleep aids like Tylenol PM and Benadryl. Instead, talk to the doctor about using Trazadone, a drug often prescribed by physicians for sleep disruption in dementia patients. Also, my husband's primary care doctor suggested we use Medisave Canada, the Canadian universal drug store, to purchase our medications. They take approximately one to three weeks to ship the medication, so you will need to plan ahead.

When taking medication is a problem, try the following:

- Use a pill cutter or crusher (if the medication allows for this).
- Request medication in liquid form.
- Add medications to ice cream, cottage cheese, yogurt, beverages, pudding, baby food... anything the patient likes and will consume.

Be aware that the doctor's nurse or secretary may put up a roadblock between you and the physician. Taking a message and not returning your phone call is unacceptable. Don't give up. If necessary, use my trick: deception.

For more medication resources, see Appendix C. A sample medication chart is located in Appendix B.

Music and Activities

Research suggests that stimulating the brain using music therapy may decrease agitation and calm patients suffering from dementia. Every case is different, but in ours, music was unquestionably a useful distraction.

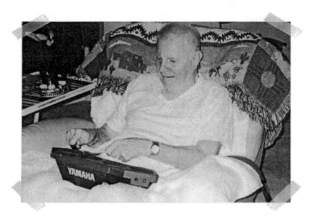

Red loved his portable drum set courtesy of the neighbors. We gave him spoons to beat the drums because they were easier to hold onto than sticks.

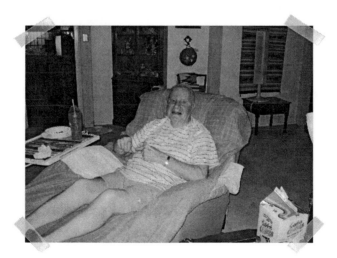

Thirty pounds heavier in early 2006.

Experiment…See what works for you and your loved one. Keep in mind that in time, focusing will be difficult and the patient's attention span will diminish.

Here is a list of activities to help you get started:

- Watching TV
- Sights & Sounds of Nature DVDs, beautiful landscape and music
- Generational movies
- Arts and crafts
- Puzzles
- Looking at family photo albums
- Musical DVDs
- Helping with household tasks
- Manicure
- Pedicure
- Massage
- Brushing, combing hair
- Playing with baby dolls
- Scrapbooking

I found a couple of handbooks on Amazon.com called: *Montessori-Based Activities for Persons with Dementia*, by Cameron J. Camp and Jennifer Bush. The handbooks were written for use with people suffering from Alzheimer's disease and similar disorders.

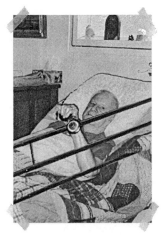

Nighttime

When Red was still responsive, we attached a horn to his bed so he could get our attention. It worked well for several months and he loved the noise.

After I moved to another room, I purchased a standard baby monitor so I could hear if he was having any problems. As the dementia progressed, I felt more secure using the camera and screen monitor mentioned in a previous chapter.

Pain Assessment

Managing pain is difficult and frequently goes untreated in dementia patients. Often patients are unable to communicate, and they may not even recognize their pain due to language deficits that can occur in the late stage of dementia.

In the early and middle stage of dementia, my husband either overreacted to pain or his perception of pain was magnified. He screamed like a little girl... my own little drama queen. Late stage, his pain reaction time was very long, from seconds to as much as a minute. This was a result of the deterioration or atrophy of his brain; in other words, progression.

As a prophylactic pain and agitation measure, we administered liquid Tylenol every four to six hours on a daily basis in late-stage dementia. We noticed almost instant pain relief and increased awareness. While administering medication at any stage, be observant.

Refer to Appendix B for a copy of the Pain Assessment in Advanced Dementia (PAINAD) Scale. This chart is especially helpful if the patient is mute.

Placement in Long-Term Care

Before placing your loved one in a facility, consider adult daycare or respite care to give yourself a breather. This may give you some extra strength to continue caregiving and reflect more clearly about admitting your loved one into a facility. If the patient is isolated in your home, a good facility can be an excellent social stimulus in addition to providing specialized care.

Keeping your loved one at home is not always possible. Late-stage dementia requires 24-hour care. This may be the point in time when you consider placing your loved one in a facility. If the following circumstances occur at any point in the disease's progression, a facility becomes a must:

- Your loved one becomes physically abusive to you or is a danger to himself or herself.

- You can no longer cope with the physical or mental demands of caregiving.
- You have medical problems of your own.

Several options are available for long-term dementia care: board and care homes, assisted living facilities, and nursing homes. Researching your options is time-consuming, confusing, and frustrating. Ask your physician, friends, or family members to help you out.

When I felt I could no longer manage my husband at home, I toured numerous facilities in Arizona and California. The price range, accommodations, smell, size, activities, and patients varied considerably. Tell me, why does a dementia patient need access to an Olympic-size swimming pool, and why would you want to pay for this wasted feature? Don't get wowed into paying for all the little extras that your loved one will never use. Think about what is most important to your loved one's health, safety, and well-being. For a price, a facility is easy to find; choosing one that fits your needs, however, requires that you do your homework.

Routine

A daily routine will keep the patient better oriented, reduce frustration, and help maintain patient independence. Create a daily schedule for eating, sleeping, bathing, dressing, and exercise. I planned our schedule around my husband's long-standing habits. As he progressed, I followed his lead. This way, he felt more in control and fewer meltdowns occurred.

Decision-making and recollection are not a dementia patient's strong points. Initially, I used a large calendar to record daily activities and appointments. With Red's recall and comprehension loss, I tried to make each day more manageable by laying out Red's clothing, simplifying his hair style, making his choices for him, taking him to the toilet every two hours, providing easy-to-eat food, and leaving his toothbrush and toothpaste on the counter.

Skin Care

I continued to take Red to the dermatologist knowing he had some nasty basal cell skin cancers. After the visits became too much for him, the doctor suggested I treat Red with a prescription cream. In addition, hospice provided us with an air mattress to prevent bed sores. A fellow caregiver shared a bed sore home remedy with me: Mix Iodine with Maalox to make a light chocolate liquid and apply to the affected area on the skin. Apparently, this creates a drying solution, especially when used with a heat lamp.

Stool and Urine Samples

Periodically, the doctor required a stool and urine

specimen. Inevitably, Red would relieve himself as we walked in the doctor's office. That being the case, we rung his diaper out in a sterile container for the perfect, fresh specimen.

If you need a stool specimen and one is currently available, snap on the rubber gloves, take a swipe, turn the glove inside out, and place it into a sealable plastic bag. Voila! No muss, and no fuss. Keep the specimen refrigerated to ensure freshness.

Swallowing Difficulty

Late stage patients will pocket their food in their cheeks rather than swallow it. Put a disposable glove on and insert your finger into his or her cheek to dislodge the food. After every two bites of food, give your loved one a sip of water. It helps to dissolve the food, making bites easier to swallow. Remember, don't put your fingers between his or her teeth, or you'll likely be bitten.

Artificial saliva may help if the mouth is dry; you can also spray small amounts of water in your loved one's mouth. After a certain point, dementia patients choke on everything, so don't force food. It can cause the patient to aspirate, meaning he or she has accidentally sucked food particles or fluids into his or her lungs, which can lead to more serious problems like pneumonia. Eventually, the patient's entire food intake may need to be the consistency of pudding.

Telephones

My husband racked up hundreds of dollars in long-distance phone calls trying to get his driver's license back while I was still working outside the home. Phone solicitors knew our phone number by heart and called on a daily basis for a friendly chat and for an invitation over to our house to sell their wares. I paid Qwest, in Arizona, an extra seven dollars a month for a No Solicitation message that automatically played when someone called our home. Unfortunately, this service may not be available in all states.

Telling Time

In the early stage of dementia, my husband was creative and resourceful, even finding new ways to tell time. Some patients may establish the time of day according to their favorite television shows, and mark the days of the week on a calendar. Even so, they may not have any idea what month it is or the name of the day.

Red would inspect the wall clock, and then put a large X on each day of the week on the erasable calendar to keep track of his imaginary schedule. He could not process time or the month as a whole, but even so, this daily routine gave him some degree of comfort.

Working after Diagnosis

Working has likely been a part of your loved one's routine for many years. Everyone needs to feel useful and productive. It is possible for a dementia patient to continue to work, so long as he or she still has language comprehension, lacks behavioral issues, and isn't a danger to himself or others. If a job is still within their capabilities, dementia patients will maintain a sense of self-worth and simultaneously stimulate their brains.

In 1996, the city of Phoenix began a job training program for disabled adults called Clear Path. The program was built around individual abilities. Check with your local Parks and Recreation Department, Department of Rehabilitation Services, library, church, or senior center about possible job opportunities for your loved one.

My husband bagged groceries for about a year at the local grocery store. He was paid minimum wage and was happy as a clam. When his supervisors feared he might lock himself in the freezer, they let him go.

Take Care of Yourself

Find a way to keep your appointment with the masseuse or your tee time at the golf course. In other words, preserve the parts of your own life that bring you happiness. If you really feel like you cannot leave your home, find people who will come to you. For example, your hairdresser may not think twice about coming to your home to cut and color your hair. The services are out there, you just need to ask.

Remember, "Don't sweat the small stuff!" You will save yourself a lot of grief if you let go, try not to control every situation, and take it one day at a time.

The best advice I received as a dementia caregiver was from Hospice of the Valley in Phoenix, Arizona. In order to minimize undesirable behaviors, "Anticipate and fulfill unmet basic needs."

"Yesterday's the past, tomorrow's the future, but today is a gift. That's why it's called the present."
—Bill Keane

SAFE KEEPING

Virginia Pasquarelli

When I was very young
My mother held me in her arms
And whispered, "Dearest one
I'll keep you safe from harm."

I was too young to understand
Every word she would say,
But the love in her voice
Comforted me every day.

When I learned to walk
She held my hand
And lent her strength
So I could stand.

A lifetime is short;
I grew older; so did she
Until the day came where
It was she that needed me.

She could barely walk
So I held her hand
And lent her my strength
So she could stand.

When she was very old,
I held her in my arms
And whispered, "Dearest one
I'll keep you safe from harm."

She was too old to understand
Every word that I said
But the love in my voice
Spoke to her instead.

At the end I held her
As she'd once held me
And I whispered, "Dearest one,
Have a safe journey."

CHAPTER FOUR

Safety

I employed aides, joined a dementia support group, got organized, and thought I was prepared for the challenge ahead. In spite of doing all of this, I was not ready for what was to come.

This chapter focuses on my challenge to keep Red safe, and the deception tactics I used to ward off danger, embarrassment, and pain. Out of necessity, I became incredibly successful at lying on a daily basis. Dishonesty and distraction has its rewards when caring for a dementia patient; namely, reducing patient agitation and caregiver stress.

Anticipate as best you can, and prepare yourself, your home, and your loved one for the worst. Focus on prevention. You cannot predict what the next second, minute, hour, or day has in store for you. Think of the patient as a toddler, and childproof your home. For my husband's safety, we transformed into conjoined twins.

Obtain referrals from your local Alzheimer's Association or Area Agency on Aging to evaluate the safety of your home. I had a local senior foundation assess our home and install grab bars for a very small price.

The National Institute on Aging has created an exceptional comprehensive room-by-room home safety list. Please use the information provided in *Appendix C* and make that phone call for a free home safety brochure.

Alarms, Gates, and Locks

I recommend fully childproofing your home. Part of this process requires that you install wireless magnetic locks with an alarm on all doors and windows. Make sure the locks are above or below your loved one's reach.

- Consolidate all soaps, cleaning supplies, and medications in locked cabinets.
- Put up tall pet gates to keep your loved one out of the kitchen when burns become a potential risk.
- I had a fence and childproof gate built around our home to keep Red from wandering off. With a doctor's prescription, I was able to write it off on my taxes.

- Place a motion detector with an indoor alarm a few steps from the front gate.
- Install childproof doorknobs. These plastic knob covers have to be squeezed in order to open the door.

My husband was intelligent, stubborn, obstinate, and resourceful. Unfortunately, I did not give him enough credit and learned many valuable lessons too late. We all suffered due to my inexperience. If you are not fully prepared, don't fret. Learn from your mistakes. And remember, gates and locks do not replace the need to be observant at all times.

Backup Plan

During my time as a caregiver, I broke three ribs, required shoulder and cataract surgery, my back went out, and a family member passed away. What was I to do with Red during these unexpected emergencies?

Recruit a trustworthy family member, friend, or homecare aide to take over when caregiver emergencies occur. It is always more convenient if you can keep your loved one at home, but there are other options available as well. Many long-term care facilities provide respite care and charge by the night. However, all health care facilities and programs require a great deal of patient information before the drop-off, leading to a lot of time-consuming paperwork. So, it's important to anticipate your needs and plan ahead. Tour the whole facility as well. Your eyes and nose may make the decision for you.

Another long-term care option is a dementia board and care residential home. They offer a bed, meals, and 24-hour supervision. Generally, they will only admit patients who do not need 24-hour medical care. Every state has its own set of standards and regulations. I would never have placed my husband in a board and care facility without shining recommendations and positive unannounced visits. In my opinion, only experienced nursing homes can offer skilled medical care appropriate for a dementia patient

Bathroom Safety

The bathroom will be the most utilized, dangerous, and time-consuming area for patients and caregivers, especially as the dementia progresses.

- Install grab bars on the inside and outside of the bathtub or shower.
- Use skid-proof bathmats in the drying area to avoid slipping.
- Make sure the shower or bathtub surface is skid-proof.
- If needed, use a bathing chair or bench with rubber non-skid tips.

- Turn down the temperature on the water heater. Initially, your loved one may try and bathe himself or herself. He or she could be severely burned if he forgets which way to turn the hot and cold knobs.
- Place all cleaning products in a lockable cabinet.

Bedroom Safety

Bed rails can pose significant safety risks when not installed properly. If the railing spaces are too far apart, a patient could very easily get his or her leg or head caught between the railings and suffocate, or end up with a severe fracture. We also had the bed rails unlatch and land on our feet. If possible, place one side of the bed against the wall and use mesh baby rails on the exposed side of the bed.

If you've ordered a hospital bed, have the deliverymen show you how to operate the bed properly. Never assume the new bed is in working order. I sent back a couple that were defective.

Depression

Alzheimer's research verifies that there is a strong correlation between dementia and depression, in some cases one being confused with the other. A job loss, memory loss, and constant confusion left my husband with his head in his hands. One day he wept and told me he was better off dead. If the patient talks about suicide, run—don't walk—and get your loved one to a doctor.

Driver's License

Dr. Allen Dobbs, professor emeritus at the University of Alberta, stated that people suffering from dementia and still driving, is a very serious problem all over North America. His statistics reveal that:

- 30-40% of dementia sufferers drive regularly;
- 40-50% have a crash within a few years of diagnosis;
- 80% of those who have a crash continue to drive;
  - 40% of these have at least one more crash;
- 25% of those asked to stop driving by law are still on the roads.

It is my belief that the family or legal guardian of a dementia patient has a moral obligation to have the patient's driver's license revoked. This will put a strain on your relationship with your loved one, but this too will pass. By putting off the inevitable, your family risks losing everything, including the lives of others. Laws differ from state to state. For instance, California physicians are required by law to report dementia-related disorders and illnesses that may result in a lapse of consciousness. Contact your local DMV to have a professional evaluate the patient's driving skills.

My husband fought relentlessly to retain his independence via his driver's license. Our primary care physician told my spouse in 1998 and again in 2001 that he should no longer get behind the wheel of a car (or, in Red's case, the cockpit of an airplane). It was a battle that included me, my husband, his physician, and the court system. I had assumed, incorrectly, that our state law required Red's primary care physician to notify the Department of Motor Vehicles of his neurological illness. Instead, the responsibility fell on me, his primary caregiver and guardian. Being the bad guy was not a role I cherished. I feared losing my husband's trust, making a horrible situation even worse. Thankfully, in 2001, our neuropsychologist submitted a letter to the Department of Motor Vehicles without hesitation, stating that Red had been diagnosed with a progressive, incurable, neurological disorder. It was her medical opinion that he was a danger to himself and others and that his license should be revoked.

Within several weeks, Red received a letter from the Department of Motor Vehicles stating that his driver's license was suspended. The DMV gave him the option of fighting the revocation order in court. By this time, he had lost the ability to read and comprehend. Not having mastered the fine art of deception just yet, I read him the letter as it was written. Guess what? Of course, he wanted his day in court. After telling the judge about his 2,000-year-old car, the verdict was obvious.

Initially, my husband was able to dig up the car keys. The fact that his license was revoked was meaningless to him. For this reason, it is imperative that you make it impossible for your loved one to access these keys, whether that means you wear the keys around your neck, disable the vehicle battery, or sell the car.

Until my husband threw in the towel, he continued to try and unlock my car with a variety of implements, including a screwdriver, hammer, saw, and gardening tools. No wonder I put on thirty pounds! This is another reason why I suggest keeping all such tools, along with any type of sharp object, under lock and key.

Lastly, alert your neighbors: During this time, Red would often wave down cars in his attempt to hitchhike from our driveway. Visitors to our home were instructed to lock their car doors and hide their keys as well. Red was famous for asking if he could borrow their cars or hop into the passenger side for a ride.

Eating and Drinking

Your local poison control and non-emergency fire and police department phone numbers should be accessible, in large print, next to the telephone.

My husband would consume anything and everything, including seashells, candles, cat food, dog food, hair tonic, checkbook registries, and dish-washing liquid. Even standing right next to him, he would wolf down anything within reach before I had a chance to remove it. Yet again, the importance of a lock and key.

Emergency Room Visits

The majority of emergency room physicians and nurses I encountered were not well-informed or dementia-friendly. You must be assertive to get proper care for your loved one.

One especially disturbing incident took place at an Emergency Room in California. My husband was visibly weak and dehydrated from persistent vomiting and diarrhea. The ambulance arrived and rushed him to the emergency room. I explained the situation and day's events to the hospital staff. I told them that I was his wife and legal guardian and that he was demented and might need to be restrained. He was frightened, agitated, and just felt rotten. The facility did not have or take the time to properly assess the situation, regardless of my adamant vocal concerns. He did need an IV but the hospital staff would not restrain him. Restraining policies differ from facility to facility. The legalese and semantics of the current laws applied to restraint are very confusing and difficult to interpret. Bottom line: Safety intervention is left to the discretion of the attending physician or hospital staff member. A decision to restrain a patient could present a substantial legal and liability risk to the facility. In this instance, I believe this facility made the wrong choice, compromising our safety as well as my husband's. Our caregiver and I had to hold down both of his arms to prevent him from pulling out the IV needle. Five minutes later, we noticed his left arm was swelling. They had missed his vein and all the saline was pumping into his arm. One of the nurses corrected the problem while we were still restraining him, but all in all, it was a very bad experience.

Falling

Remove anything and everything your loved one might trip or stumble over. In the event the patient does fall, do not attempt to lift him or her by yourself. Call your non-emergency fire department for assistance or 911.

Statistics show that 40 to 60% of dementia patients will fall at least once. Difficulty with balance, medical issues, medicinal side effects, and the environment can all contribute to this challenge.

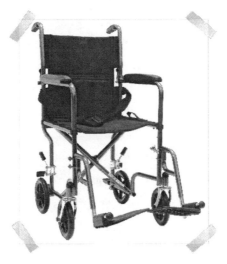

Light-Weight Folding Transport Chair

I found this product to be invaluable when balance was an issue or when I was concerned about Red injuring himself. The product is foldable, inexpensive, and lightweight. I purchased this item gently used from a medical supply store.

Kitchen

This was our hot spot in the early stages of dementia. Almost everything in our kitchen endangered my husband. Start out by removing, hiding, or locking up anything sharp and installing gates at the kitchen entrance to prevent your loved one from sneaking in without your knowledge.

Medications

Many over-the-counter and prescription medications will do more harm than good and should not be given to a dementia patient. Never give your loved one any medication without first checking with your doctor, preferably a neurologist. Keep all medications locked away.

Adverse side effects are possible with any medication. As a caregiver, monitor and report anything unusual to the physician. The physician should also warn you of any potential side effects and order periodic blood work-ups. If they don't, ask them to.

Passenger Seat Precautions

There is a possibility it will not be safe to have your loved one as a passenger in your car without taking precautions. I realized I could not drive alone with Red in the car when he grabbed the steering wheel and opened the car door while we were on the freeway. After this unpleasant incident, Red was only allowed to ride in the backseat of the car on a waterproof pad (in case of an accident). I engaged the car door baby locks, window locks, and fastened his seatbelt upside down so he could not unbuckle it. He actually figured out how to roll the window down and open the door from the outside. The solution? Have an additional caregiver sit in the front passenger seat or in the back seat with the patient to stop any unwanted activity.

Patient's Wallet or Purse

One of my husband's security blankets was his wallet. When I felt he could no longer be trusted with finances, I substituted everything in his wallet with dollar bills, an Alzheimer's photo ID card, his insurance cards, and emergency phone numbers. Red never knew the difference. Of course, this substitution took place in the dead of night. Deception takes effort and forethought.

Strangers

The emotional and financial impact of dementia creates a world of susceptibility. When deceitful people discover you are caring for a patient with an incurable disorder, they may congregate on your doorstep. Caregivers beware! Be wary of anyone who offers you anything too good to be true. Form a trusted circle of friends and family. Unfortunately, you and your loved one are now very vulnerable.

During the last year of my husband's life, out of the blue, a long-time neighbor began walking his dog daily through our yard. According to him, I was the most congenial woman on the block. That's nice. Little did I realize he was appraising our homestead as a potential sale. He began putting his business card in our mailbox and calling with offers in an attempt to purchase our home. I reminded him my husband was not dead yet. From that day forward, he has not set one foot on our property.

Wandering

Statistically, more than half of all patients diagnosed with dementia will wander. This is why it is crucial to register with the MedicAlert + Safe Return Program. Purchase a Safe Return bracelet or necklace for yourself, your loved one, and any additional care-givers. The jewelry contains a toll-free emergency phone number along with the patient's medical conditions, allergies, and identification number. One phone call activates the 24-hour nationwide support network. In addition, if you are in an accident, physi-cians, police, and paramedics will use the informa-tion on the jewelry to alert the network, who will locate your loved one and make sure they are safe. It is a small price to pay for peace of mind.

My husband did not want to wear his ID bracelet. Although there is a safety clasp, he still managed to get it off. I thought he might cut his hand off to remove his bracelet. I even presented the ID bracelet to him as a gift and showed him that I had one as well. Didn't work. I had his doctor give it back to him as an award of valor. Didn't work. I finally attached it to his shoe-lace, luckily without an argument.

To enroll in the program or for suggestions on how to get your loved one to wear his or her ID jewelry, go to http://www.medicalert.org or call 1-888-633-4298.

The lesson of this chapter? Consider everything a potential—and probable—hazard. Dementia patients can be large, strong, fearless toddlers. They will not learn the hard way, you will.

Take Care of Yourself

If you are so anxious or agitated that you cannot focus or sleep at night, you may want to consider anti-anxiety medication or antidepressants. Do not be embarrassed or ashamed for needing your own medical support to keep your sanity. You are beginning a new life as a caregiver and it is important that you stay physically and emotionally resilient.

Many physicians and service organizations have labeled the stress on a caregiver's body, mind, and spirit, "caregiver syndrome." The unrelenting 24-hour care of individuals with a chronic illness also leads to additional financial, physical, and emotional responsibility.

In my opinion, our country has yet to step up to the plate to recognize the millions of caregivers abruptly entrusted with this responsibility. According to the National Alliance for Caregiving and Evercare, in-home caregivers save our health care system billions of dollars, while risking their own health in return. Caregivers become so absorbed in their new role that they often do not realize they are neglecting themselves. Losing interest in the activities you once took pleasure in is a sure sign you need to make a doctor's appointment for yourself.

GIVING
Virginia Pasquarelli

Being the one
Who cares day after day
Can be tiring and frightening
When we don't know the way.

There isn't a manual,
No expert to call
Who can say, "Do not worry,
I know it all."

So we learn about caring,
By doing and trying
To make life bearable
For a loved one who is dying.

There are often days
We aren't really sure
If we can bear the burden
A single minute more.

But some days we know
That we've gotten it right.
By the peace on their face,
By a smile that's bright.

Or simply by knowing
That all that we do
Is just giving back
The love they gave, too.

CHAPTER FIVE

Late-Stage Dementia

As the final stage of dementia gains momentum, this progressive, incurable disorder requires complete care 24-hours a day, 7 days a week. Your loved one's body will begin to shut down, and he or she will become dependent on your unconditional love and commitment for every aspect of life.

Dementia progresses differently in every individual, making it impossible to predict how long your loved one will live. Red required over a year of end-stage care while other patients may require only a few days. According to http://www.helpguide.org, the average duration can be from one to three years.

Although your loved one may not be able to speak, his or her emotional memories may linger. Create a relaxed atmosphere to preserve his dignity and well-being through his final chapter of life. Your caring presence, voice, and physical contact will be an immense comfort to your loved one.

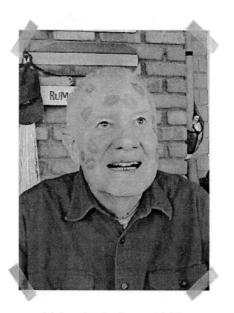

Valentine's Day, 2005

Additional problems and concerns will surface in the late stage of dementia: How much longer will my loved one live? Should I continue administering medication? How do I know if he or she is in pain?

If you have chosen to keep your loved one at home during this stage, work with family members, physicians, and hospice to address your questions and concerns. Above all, be prepared in every sense of the word for that final moment by having all arrangements ready well in advance. To help you prepare, I've compiled a list of medical complications and other concerns below. The list appears in alphabetical order by topic.

Advance Directives

Advance directives are legal instructions that document end-of-life care choices. Advance directives commonly consist of three official directives:

1. *Living Will* – instructs physicians and relatives how we wish to be treated if we become incapacitated by illness or injury.

2. *Durable Power of Attorney* – designates another person to act on the patient's behalf, in the event that the individual becomes disabled or incapacitated.

3. *Durable Health Care Power of Attorney* – appoints a person to make medical decisions on your behalf when you are no longer able to make medical decisions for yourself.

It is very important to obtain advance directives for patients with dementia while they are in the early stages, still cognizant and able to sign their names. If your loved one is no longer capable of making decisions, the family is responsible for making all end-of-life resolutions. With advance directives in place, family members are relieved of the pressure and guilt.

Forms can be obtained from your doctor, attorney, or your State Department on Aging. Have your doctor or attorney review the directives to make sure they correctly communicate your intentions. Once notarized, distribute copies to family members, physicians, and your attorney.

A Do Not Resuscitate (DNR) order is a written document that states you do not want to be resuscitated if your breathing and heartbeat stop. In some states, if you do not have a DNR, firefighters and paramedics are required by law to transport the patient to the emergency room for treatment. Check with your elder law attorney or hospice in regards to the laws in your state to assist you with your decision.

I kept my husband's DNR in plain sight on our refrigerator. I did not want his final moments to be in unfamiliar surroundings such as the emergency room or hospital.

A DNR may be obtained by the patient's health care power of attorney, attending physician, hospital, or hospice. DNR guidelines vary from state to state, especially regarding out-of-hospital (ambulance) care. Most states have a standardized form varying in wording and color. If the DNR order is not written on the approved state form, it will not be honored. DNR orders are one of the many services that hospice programs provide; some may even require them as a condition of enrollment.

Advance directives are legally valid in the United States as soon as they are signed in front of the required witnesses. You do not need a lawyer to fill out advance directives, but I would recommend having one regardless. It is also important to comply with your state's law, as they do differ state by state.

Approaching Death

The signs of imminent death will vary from person to person. It may help to understand the normal changes that take place during this process and how best to respond.

Breathing Changes and Congestion

Breathing may become shallow, uneven, fast, or unusually slow. Changes may cause a moaning-like sound when individuals exhale. Congestion is common, and is caused by fluid build-up in the lungs. To avoid choking, elevate your loved one's head using pillows, or turn his or her head to the side.

Biot's Respiration occurs when breathing is irregular with periods of apnea usually equal in rate and depth.

Cheyne–Stokes Respiration, also known as the death rattle, defined by Hospice Foundation of America: "Likely just hours from death; breathing changes from a normal rate and rhythm to a new pattern of several rapid breaths followed by a period of no breathing. These patterns are very common and indicate decrease in circulation in the internal organs."

Decreased Food and Fluid Intake

Your loved one will begin eating and drinking less. As a result, he or she will lose weight and strength. Never force food or fluids, and keep his or her mouth and lips moist using wet swabs, ice chips, and lip balm to prevent cracking and dryness.

Increased Sleep

The patient may spend more time sleeping at the end of life or retreat by closing his or her eyes. This natural change is due in part to changes in metabolism. Keep in mind that the patient can still hear what is being said during this time. Does he or she comprehend? I witnessed two lucid moments during Red's late stage so I did not take any chances.

Restlessness

Agitation and repetitive motions are common. He or she may groan, scream, or mumble. Comfort him or her by holding his hand or gently massaging his forehead. Softly reassure him, or play his favorite music.

Skin Tone

The color of the patient's skin may change. This is a normal sign that his or her blood circulation is being reserved for the most crucial organs, decreasing the flow to his extremities.

Swallowing and Choking

Swallowing and choking problems are common at this stage. Proper positioning can reduce choking. Make sure the patient is seated at a 90-degree angle. Sit at the patient's eye level when feeding him or her, and do not put too much food in his mouth at once. Let your loved one enjoy his meal by allowing him as much time as necessary. Keep the patient in an upright position for at least half an hour after eating, and cleanse the mouth of debris after each meal.

Temperature

Your loved one's arms and legs may become progressively cooler or warmer to the touch. Warm him or her if he appears cold, but do not use an electric blanket and risk overheating him or burning his delicate skin.

Urine Decrease

Due to the decline in fluid intake, urine output decreases and becomes more concentrated, turning the color of tea.

Autopsy

You may choose to have an autopsy completed on your loved one. During an autopsy, a pathologist performs a medical exam of the body to provide answers regarding the nature of the person's illness or cause of death. In the case of dementia, the brain is removed and analyzed to provide an accurate diagnosis. However, the brain tissue will not be studied for research purposes. Upon completion of the autopsy, you should receive a written report that describes the findings.

If cognizant, the patient should make his or her preferences known regarding an autopsy when filling out his advance directives.

Brain Donation

Unlike an autopsy, brain donation requires removing brain tissue for the purpose of study. Brain donation needs to be planned months in advance, typically by a qualified patient enrolling in a clinical research program. These studies require all of the patient's medical records in addition to further examination and testing at the medical research facility. Prior to death, the program's researchers will provide you with comprehensive instructions, phone numbers, and advice to assist you at this difficult time. If you are enrolled in a clinical research program, there is seldom any cost to the family aside from transportation.

If you are donating your loved one's brain, organs, or tissue, notify the selected research facility of any sudden decline in his or her health. Within several months of death you should receive a written report detailing the nature and diagnosis of your loved one's dementia. It is important to keep in mind that researchers cannot find a cure unless we all consider participating in a brain donation program.

Comfort Care

Ask hospice to assist you in providing comfort care for your loved one at this stage in his or her life. Hospice services provide a wonderful support system that includes social workers, pastoral and bereavement counselors, nurses, aides, and volunteers.

Comfort care focuses on the following goals:

- Relieve the patient's pain and suffering.
- Provide the patient with emotional, mental, and spiritual well-being.
- Respect the patient's independence and dignity.
- Support family members during and after death.
- Provide references for local hospice care facilities where the patient will be most comfortable.

Eating and Feeding

Most, if not all, late-stage dementia patients lose weight. Your loved one may have forgotten how to chew or swallow, he or she may no longer recognize food as nourishment, or he may just not want to eat.

When your loved one develops swallowing difficulties, it may help to purée his or her favorite foods. I incorporated nutritional shakes as well. The thick consistency is perfect, they are high in calories, and they taste good.

The Dysphagia Cookbook by Elayne Achilles has some very good guidelines for patients with swallowing difficulties. The recipes are easy and nutritionally balanced for every phase of dysphagia. The cookbook may be purchased at Amazon.com.

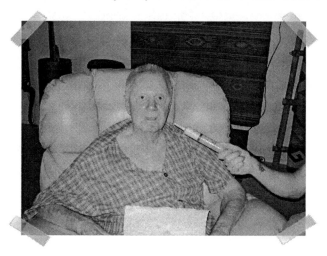

Thanksgiving Day, 2006. Puréed Thanksgiving dinner served with a 6-ounce food syringe. It smelled just like a turkey dinner.

We tried to make mealtime fun to persuade my husband to eat. We used old dishcloths and cut a hole for his head instead of buying adult bibs. Many small meals a day seemed to work better than three larger ones. We always kept a snack plate next to his chair. The more advanced the dementia, the softer and smaller the snacks must be. As Red started to become disinterested in eating, we fed him foods high in calories and fat to prevent weight-loss. Eventually, he lost interest in eating altogether.

Hydration is also a major issue, especially in the later stages of dementia. The brain may not be regulating the thirst reflex or body temperature. Encourage, but do not force food or liquid intake. If your loved one can't use a straw, try a baby sippy cup.

Feeding Tubes

Another difficult decision to make is whether you want to use a feeding tube. The answer to this question may be as easy as referring to your loved one's advance directives.

Hospice offered to insert a feeding tube into my husband three months before the end of his life. He was in the advanced stage of dementia in an infant state. Did I want to prolong his suffering? Would this procedure enhance his quality of life? The answer was a definite no.

As you make your decision, keep in mind that there is a certain amount of discomfort and risk associated with a feeding tube, which can lead to any of the following complications:

- Discomfort at the time of insertion
- Diarrhea
- Infection, skin irritation, or bedsores at tube site
- Pneumonia (as many as 50% of patients aspirate stomach contents into their lungs)
- Congestive heart failure caused by excess fluid in the lungs

If you are forced to make this very personal choice, please give it a lot of thought and discuss the pros and cons with other family members as well as your physician before making your decision.

I knew Red was not hungry or thirsty in the final stage of his life, but the act of hand-feeding him brought us even closer together. I know my love, care, and touch meant the world to him.

Hospice

You will need your physician to request and recommend a hospice care agency. The agency will then send out a representative to evaluate your loved one. They will either recommend a local hospice care facility or provide you with everything you need, including medication, to keep your loved one comfortable at home. As of this writing, hospice will bill Medicare if your loved one is over the age of sixty-five.

Hospice nurses are typically on call around the clock. If you ever run into an unbearable situation, do not hesitate to call.

Pain Management

According to most pain and palliative centers, in an advanced dementia patient, pain recognition and response weakens due to damage to specific parts of the brain; therefore, his or her pain may go untreated. If your loved one is mute, focus on body language, facial expressions, acute agitation, and verbal cues (such as moaning) to determine if he or she is in pain.

If you think your loved one might be in pain, tell your hospice nurse immediately. Hospice supplied me with a topical pain medication that was both an anti-inflammatory as well as a muscle relaxant.

Refer to Appendix B for the Pain Assessment in Advanced/Non-verbal Dementia (PAINAD) Scale.

Seizures/Tremors/Spasms

My husband had involuntary movement in both arms, hands, tongue, and lower jaw for several years. Agitation or anxiety made his tremors more violent.

While researching this issue, I learned that dementia may damage or destroy parts of the brainstem, resulting in an increase in the chance for involuntary movements such as seizures or tremors. Some psychotropic medications, such as Haldol, may also be a factor thanks to a side effect called dyskinesia, which can create permanent distortions in voluntary movement.

Hospice and I believe that my husband's involuntary movements were a combination of issues stemming from the damage caused by the progression of his dementia. Our best guess was a neurological condition defined as myoclonus. The National Institute of Neurological Disorders and Stroke describes it as,"sudden, involuntary jerking of a muscle or group. Myoclonic twitches or jerks usually are caused by sudden muscle contractions, called positive myoclonus, or by muscle relaxation, called negative myoclonus. Myoclonic jerks may occur alone or in sequence, in a pattern or without pattern. They may occur infrequently or many times each minute. Myoclonus sometimes occurs in response to an external event or when a person attempts to make a movement. The twitching cannot be controlled by the person experiencing it."

Alert your physician or hospice if you notice your loved one making involuntary movements, as this may be a precursor to a seizure or other serious problem.

Shortened Tendons

We tried reflexology, daily gentle massage with warm lotion, squeezing rubber balls—anything and everything to deter the inevitable physical response to inactivity.

The photo below of my husband's feet shows the results of a long-term sedentary lifestyle.

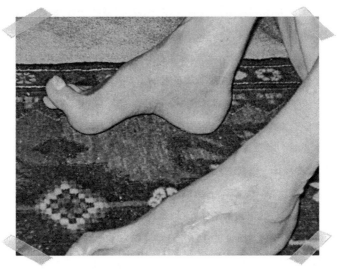

It is important to be aware of the multitude of physical and mental challenges dementia can present. The symptomology of a patient's physical and mental being is based on the specific areas of the brain that are damaged. What occurs in one patient may not occur in another patient with the same diagnosis. I knew my husband's may not be typical of all dementia patients, leading me to believe Red was stricken with several neurological problems. His brain autopsy later confirmed this to be true. There is no way to predict what direction dementia will take or brain tissue it will destroy.

Sudden Decline

I cannot tell you how many "sudden declines" I thought my husband had undergone during the progression of the beast. A few of the more discon-certing observations included acute high fevers, abrupt loss of balance, drooling, respiratory prob-lems, rapid shallow breathing, eyes focused on the ceiling, mouth open, and lethargy. Our living room looked more like a large hospital room, with Red our sole focus of attention. A camera was attached to a ceiling beam to monitor his every breath from each room in our home. Hospital bed, electric air mattress, oxygen, nebulizer, medical supplies, diapers, wet wipes, barf buckets—we were prepared for any emergency. In spite of his declining health, Red still greeted anyone who entered the room in his own sweet way. He was mute, but would smile and offer some drooled-on M&M's or crackers.

Red's rapid final decline began in October of 2006. This time he did not recover as he had so many times before. Hospice sent a pastor once a week as a comfort measure and, I suppose, as a means of preparing me for his final departure. The eternal Girl

Scout, I wrote my husband's obituary on October 24, 2006, less than 2 months before his death.

REMEMBER
Virginia Pasquarelli

Even if you've forgotten my name,
Or the nickname I always called you.
Even if you've forgotten you loved me,
I will just remember for two.

I know you don't know who I am,
When I bend to give you a kiss.
You might not shed a tear,
For the things that you will miss.

But I will miss every moment,
All the things we planned to do.
And I promise with all my heart,
I will always remember you.

CHAPTER SIX

The Final Departure

At the time of your loved one's death, ask a supportive family member or friend to come over, particularly if the death occurs at home. If your loved one is a hospice patient, immediately report the death to your hospice nurse. Hospice will come to your home and pronounce the time of death according to your recall and may assist you with important phone calls.

If you choose not to use hospice, paramedics should be called to pronounce the death. As difficult as this day will be, take comfort in knowing that your loved one is finally resting in peace.

Caregiver Grief

There is no right or wrong way to grieve. The grieving process is unique to every individual. Remember, there is no standard or correct timetable.

Common reactions to your loved one's death include:

- Anger
- Confusion
- Depression and withdrawal
- Difficulty making decisions
- Dry mouth
- Apathy
- Guilt
- Insomnia
- Loss of appetite and energy
- Nausea
- Trouble breathing

Be indulgent and patient with yourself. Allow nature to take its course without any self-induced restrictions.

Death Checklist

In the weeks leading up to Red's passing, I prepared a checklist from a combination of online resources that fit my needs. My ultimate goal was to go through this process without feeling forced to think; I correctly predicted that I would have a very difficult time focusing on anything for several weeks after that final moment.

Refer to Appendix B for a sample Checklist Following Death. If this list does not fit your individual needs, numerous other lists can be found online. The funeral home, your physician, attorney, or CPA may also have forms more suitable for your personal and financial needs.

At Peace

Wednesday began like any other day in the land of dementia. Hospice had just left. Their impression was that Red had approximately six more months to live. I wanted to believe them, but deep down I knew that was impossible. The electrician arrived early to rewire the living room to accommodate all of my husband's medical devices. Since all was stable on the home front, Michelle and I decided to run some errands together. Michelle's son, whom Red adored, would sit for the next hour so we could get a break. I should have gone with my gut feeling.

After receiving a frantic phone call at the store, we flew home at lightning speed. There he sat, finally in peace and free of pain. I can only describe my immediate reaction as denial. It couldn't be. I had left him in his recliner not half an hour ago, laughing and listening to his headphones. Even in death, he surprised me when my head was turned.

A gentle kiss verified that I had missed that final moment by seconds: his lips were still warm. December 6, 2006 at 1:39 p.m., still in his recliner, headphones blasting with the music of Pavarotti, this chapter of our lives was over. I recall having told him weeks prior that I would be all right if he wanted to go. I guess he heard me.

I had only a moment to cry before I remembered I had to call our hospice nurse, and more importantly, the University of San Francisco organ donor autopsy service, to report the death.

The University of San Francisco called the harvesting hospital and made arrangements for pick-up. We were instructed to ice the back of Red's neck near the brain stem area as a preservative measure. Several hours later, the crew from the hospital wheeled Red out the front door just as our mailman was walking up the driveway to deliver a Christmas gift that Red's caregiver had ordered for me, from my husband.

My husband's memorial was held at Fort Rosecrans National Cemetery three months later. Just moments after "Taps," we were returning to our vehicles when three Air Force jets took off from North Island as though I had planned it. Maybe Red did! I could not have asked for any better send-off for my F-100 fighter pilot.

I received the first letter from the University of Pennsylvania Medical Center on March 2, 2007. The brain autopsy examination was complete. They were now going to begin the detailed analysis of the nervous system tissue samples to determine the exact diagnosis of my husband's neurological disorder. I received their final report approximately six months later, with a reminder that "Brain donation makes possible the scientific advances necessary for establishing a definitive treatment for neurodegenerative disorders."

The University of Pennsylvania concluded that my husband had Semantic Dementia, a form of Frontal Temporal Dementia, with some Lewy Bodies present. I was not even aware that "Semantic Dementia" existed. This just goes to show how far research has come since my husband's initial diagnosis…just not far enough.

The four-year anniversary of my husband's death came and went. My eyes still well up with sadness from the loss and what was taken from both of us—nearly fifteen years of our lives. Fortunately, he was not as aware of this theft as I was, a sort of dementia bonus. At times it is difficult to look back on our amazing life together pre-dementia, because more than half of our twenty-four year marriage was spent confronting the demon.

Our experience pushed me beyond my limits and changed my life forever. I discovered I was a strong, capable, stubborn woman able to endure more than should be expected or allowed in one lifetime. I also recognized that the disorder forced me to focus on what is actually important in life: love, family, health, and laughter.

Though this book does not even scratch the surface of this dreadful disorder, it is a start. Completion of *The Journey Ahead* brings me closure, and the realization that the greatest accomplishment in my life will forever be my role as caregiver.

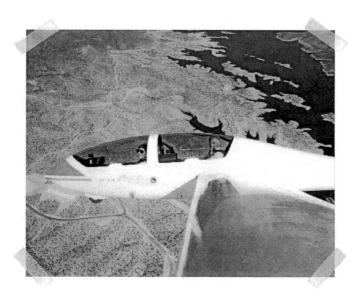

Fond Memories

APPENDIX A: *Voice of a Caregiver*

Our online caregiver support group was founded by Harv, a fellow caregiver and friend, on May 14, 2002. Our group is dementia-specific. To date, 278 of us have cared for family members, spouses, or close friends diagnosed with Primary Progressive Aphasia. This syndrome is defined by UCSF Memory and Aging Center: "PPA is caused by degeneration in the parts of the brain that control speech and language (the left, or 'dominant,' side of the brain in the frontal, temporal, and parietal regions). This type of aphasia begins gradually, with speech or language symptoms that will vary depending on the brain areas affected by the disease."

The fact that I was no longer alone in my quest for emotional support and information probably saved my life. Many of us have lost loved ones, but remain members of the group as caregivers' advocates. We whine, snivel, cry, laugh, share, brainstorm, and problem-solve.

I wanted to include quotes from my fellow caregivers to give them another voice and let you know you are not alone. My online friends will validate your feelings as a caregiver. You are overworked, undervalued, and...you are incredible.

"Damn it, is it 5 o'clock yet?"
Barb (We miss you, Mom.), 1994

"Live and die with dignity. The drugs worked for a short time, and we just toughed it out after that. When he began to sleep all the time at the end, we probably should have taken him to the hospital, but we just couldn't put him through it again. If we had, he might have lived longer. Even his neurologist at Northwestern was surprised he died when he did."

"I guess what I'm trying to say, and I know you agree, is that the caregiver knows the patient better than the doctor. They may be professionals, but we have to know when to quit."
Lorraine, 2007

"I do have regrets for not planning better and talking more about the future in the early stages of JoEllen's illness. Initially there was some thought that she had a stroke, so all the focus was on speech therapy and getting well. But by the time the first PPA diagnosis was made, her communication skills were pretty much non-existent. Our wills, POA's, health directives, etc. were all in place before her illness. But so many other things important to us—our relationship, our kids and grandkids—weren't discussed or documented in time before she became mute and unable to write. So I live with those regrets and hope that other families facing a PPA diagnosis would be forewarned to prepare early before it is too late."

"Eye exams for possible prescription change should be another must-do at an early stage. By the time of JoEllen's scheduled eye exam she was unable to help the doctor determine if a correction was needed. So now the eye exam is only to check the health of her eyes, and the idea of improving vision is no longer possible, since the refraction exam requires full cooperation of the patient."
Charlie, November 2010

"I know you feel like it is taking over your life. But, I think we have to think about this differently than we are. I think we just have to face that our loved

ones have a terrible illness that requires a lot of love, strength, patience and understanding on the part of many people to get them through in comfort and safety, as much as that is possible. No nursing home, no aide, no helper, no son, no one doctor, no one expert…no person can get our loved ones through this. It takes the biggest team we can put together, but as spouses or children who love the person like no one else involved, we'll never be able to give the job to someone else entirely. We have to make a promise to ourselves and our loved ones that we know and expect tough times ahead, and that we will rise to each frightening, exhausting, or frustrating occasion with the most love and effort we can put forth, and use every bit of help we can find on the way."
Ginny, December 2009

"Caregivers who join our online support group frequently ask, "What can we expect?" We can only tell them that little about one person's situation applies to others, except in very general terms."

"Generalities are not useful, as cases are extremely individualized. As a result, not all the symptoms or effects you may know of will apply."
Harv, January 2010

"As part of UCSF's Memory and Aging Center's long-term FTD study, JoEllen had multiple tests including MRI, fMRI, PIB Scan, eye scans, etc., etc., and yet there is no certainty that she in fact has PPA (specifically PNFA). That is one reason why it is important for research that patients donate their brains to an autopsy program so doctors can learn if their early diagnosis was correct."
Charlie, November 2010

"There are so many options in dealing with dementia, some good, and some bad. You just have to make decisions and live with them."
Charles, 2000

"It is a very difficult realization but this is a terminal disease. You need to plan for your future because eventually you will be on your own."
Mickey, May 2002

"Bottom line, each year brings a new level of coping."
Carole

"Maintain a normal life as long as you can. If there is family you want to see, places you want to go, things you want to do with your loved ones…don't wait."
Anonymous

"Someone has said this illness brings out the best and worst in people. I think we all have good and bad traits which are easy enough to tolerate when things are good, but when something bad happens, no one has the patience for it and it brings everything to the forefront."
Val

"While there is really nothing anyone can say or do that will change what we are all facing or make it go away, I think it sometimes helps to just talk and vent, and to know that there are at least some other people who truly understand--like all the people on this support site. Take care of yourself, chin up, be grateful for every tiny positive thing that you can enjoy, and just carry on day by day—that's all we can do—and on some days, it's almost enough to get you through."
Barb, November 2010

"Finding pleasure and joy is a never-ending task, just as caring for a PPA spouse is...so many people do not understand; of course, they don't have a PPA spouse!"
Lou Ann, November 2010

"My husband Tommy passed away December 19 after showing symptoms in 2005 with a diagnosis in 2008. A childhood friend, a neurologist, openly wept at the diagnosis; our family doctor flatly stated we had been dealt the shittiest hand...a ticking bomb in the brain, no cure, no biomarkers YET, no medicine, no timeline. We could certainly relate to the Pink Floyd lyric, *There's someone in my head and it's not me.* As I researched the disease and became a member of the PPA online support group, it was clear that we were in for a bumpy ride. The first posted response from all after "joining" would generally be that of a sympathetic...yet evasive we are so sorry you are part of this group...and get your legal affairs in order. As the years would go on through workshops and Internet communication we would all become a global family watching our loved ones live out a disaster."

"Facing a terminal illness was met with every bit of gumption we could muster up. Tommy was part of a research study funded by the National Institutes of Health, at Northwestern University and participated in NOVA graduate student programs for communication disorders. This was not to be a gloomy ride, but a path to another opportunity. Tommy's brain was harvested immediately and sent to Northwestern. We had made that conscious decision long before the going got tough. Our family dynamic has changed, but not the joie de vivre he left within each of us who were fortunate to know a fun, sweet, kind, tall dark handsome man."

'Make it Count'… no regrets. God Bless.

"Bless you all my PPA family, I hold you all dearly in my heart as you guided me and supported each day."

Lee, December 2010

"As time has passed, I don't check this email as often as I did when I was in the midst of the struggle with Mom. I've been trying to do exactly what you wrote: 'Make it Count.' Best to you in doing that in the coming months and years. While we grieve and miss our loved ones terribly, we wouldn't be making it count if we stood still. There is more to do in this life for all of us after we've allowed ourselves time to heal."

Loveday, January 2011

"We have missed you, Derry. We miss your kindness and consideration, your friendliness and respect for everyone. We miss your intelligence and knowledge, your humor and your quick wit. We miss our problem solver and handyman. We even miss Derryisms and our "best before date" disdainer. I miss our talks, our walks, and our enjoyment together of our children, our garden and nature. I miss our love. Now I will miss seeing you. You were a good and gentle man, and you were loved truly."

Janice, January 2011

APPENDIX B: *Caregiver Tools*

Adult Daycare Center Checklist

This checklist is intended for use when selecting an adult daycare center. Complete this checklist for each facility you visit and then use this information to compare the different facilities.

Name of Facility: Date of Visit:

Address: Phone Number:

Director Name: Hours of Operation:

Basic Information	Yes	No	Comments
Is the center licensed by a state regulatory agency?	☐	☐	
How long has the center been open?	# of years:		
Is a valid license posted?	☐	☐	
Does the center have half-day program?	☐	☐	
Does the center have full-day program?	☐	☐	
Are there any age requirements?	☐	☐	

Does the center accept individuals with Alzheimer's or dementia, limited mobility, and/or incontinence?

Are special services (e.g., Alzheimer's, dementia, rehabilitation) offered?

Can the center provide care for your relative given how incapacitated he or she is?

Cost	Yes	No	Comments

What is the fee for the hours and services you need?

Are there discounts available for those with lower incomes?

What services are included in that fee?

Is a deposit required? How much?

What additional services
are available and at
what costs?

_____
_____
_____

Is any of the cost
covered by Medicare,
Medicaid, private
insurance, or other
financial aid?

☐ ☐

_____
_____
_____

Is a deposit required?
How much?

☐ ☐

_____
_____
_____

Services Provided	**Needed (L)** **Available (R)**	**Comments**
Art and crafts	☐ ☐	_____ _____
Assistance with bathing, dressing, grooming, or toileting	☐ ☐	_____ _____ _____
Dietary counseling	☐ ☐	_____ _____
Exercise	☐ ☐	_____ _____
Laundry	☐ ☐	_____ _____

Meals at center ☐ ☐ _____
_____

Medical assessment ☐ ☐ _____
_____

Medical treatment ☐ ☐ _____
_____

Medicine management ☐ ☐ _____
_____

Music therapy ☐ ☐ _____
_____

Occupational therapy ☐ ☐ _____
_____

Physical therapy ☐ ☐ _____
_____

Recreation ☐ ☐ _____
_____

Social services ☐ ☐ _____
_____

Speech therapy ☐ ☐ _____
_____

Transportation to the center ☐ ☐ _____
_____

Transportation (other) ☐ ☐ _____
_____

Activities	Yes	No	Comments
Are activity schedules varied and based on resident's interests?	☐	☐	_____
Are activity schedules varied and based on resident's interests?	☐	☐	_____
Do residents provide input or help plan activities?	☐	☐	_____
Is reading assistance available?	☐	☐	_____
Are there protected/ enclosed areas for residents with dementia?	☐	☐	_____
Who develops and supervises recreational activities? What is their background?			_____

Standards of Care	Yes	No	Comments
Can the participant bring a caregiver with him/her to the center?	☐	☐	_____ _____ _____
Is there a separate place for sick persons to sit or sleep isolated from the other participants?	☐	☐	_____ _____ _____
What is the procedure if a medical problem occurs?			_____ _____ _____
How does staff handle difficult behavior?			_____ _____ _____
What is the bathroom procedure?			_____ _____ _____
Do participants have to wait if they need assistance?	☐	☐	_____ _____ _____
How is health monitored? How often?			_____ _____ _____

Participants	Yes	No	Comments
Are residents interacting with each other?	☐	☐	
What do residents like best about the facility? Least?			
What is daily life like at the center?			

Environment	Yes	No	Comments
Is the center clean, pleasant, and free of odor?	☐	☐	
Is the temperature comfortable for residents?	☐	☐	
Is the center well-lit?	☐	☐	
Are there quiet and/ or private areas for conferences or private conversations?	☐	☐	

Are noise levels
in common areas
comfortable?

□ □

_____
_____
_____

Is smoking not allowed
or is it restricted to
certain sections of the
center?

□ □

_____
_____
_____

Are furnishings
comfortable, sturdy, and
attractive?

□ □

_____
_____
_____

Are the building and
grounds well cared for
and attractive?

□ □

_____
_____
_____

Staff	**Yes**	**No**	**Comments**

Does the staff wear
name tags?

□ □

_____
_____
_____

Does the relationship
between staff and
participants appear to
be polite, warm, and
respectful?

□ □

_____
_____
_____

Is the staff friendly, considerate, and helpful to you?

☐ ☐ _____

If participants or staff are not native English speakers, can they communicate effectively with each other?

☐ ☐ _____

What is the staff-participant ratio?

_____

What kind of qualifications or experience does the staff have?

_____

Menus and Food   **Yes   No**   **Comments**

Does the food look and smell good?

☐ ☐ _____

Do residents have a choice of food items at each meal?

☐ ☐ _____

Are favorite foods offered?

☐ ☐ _____

Can staff help residents
eat and drink at
mealtimes if needed?

☐ ☐ _____
_____
_____

Safety and Security   Yes   No   **Comments**

Does the center meet
local, state, and federal
fire codes?

☐ ☐ _____
_____
_____

Are emergency
exits clearly
marked, accessible,
unobstructed, and easily
opened from the inside?

☐ ☐ _____
_____
_____

Are there fire safety
systems? (For example,
smoke detectors, fire
extinguishers, and
sprinklers are in each
room.)

☐ ☐ _____
_____
_____

Is there an emergency
evacuation plan? Is it
posted?

☐ ☐ _____
_____
_____

Is the center wheelchair-
accessible?

☐ ☐ _____
_____
_____

What safety measures
are in place to protect
residents from
wandering?

_____
_____
_____

Are there written
policies about what
is considered an
emergency, when 911 is
called and who decides
to call?

☐ ☐

_____
_____
_____

What happens if
the participant's
transportation home at
the end of the day is
delayed in picking up
the participant?

_____
_____
_____
_____
_____
_____

Transportation	**Yes**	**No**	**Comments**

Does the center offer
transportation for
appointments?

☐ ☐

_____
_____
_____

Are there costs
involved in using their
transportation?

☐ ☐

_____
_____
_____

Is transportation
wheelchair-accessible? ☐ ☐ _____
_____
_____

Is transportation
available for non-
medical appointments? ☐ ☐ _____
_____
_____

General rating on a scale of 1 (poor) to 5 (excellent):

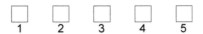

Used with permission from AGIS Network, AssistGuide Information Services, 2410 Camino Ramon, Bishop Ranch 6, Suite 343, San Ramon, CA 94583.

Toll-Free Phone Number: 1-866-511-9186, info@agis.com, Copyright 2008. All rights reserved.
http://www.agis.com

Car Tool Kit

- Air freshener
- Bottles of water and/or favorite beverages
- Emergency names and phone numbers
- Extra diapers
- Finger-food snacks
- Garbage bags
- Tissues for drooling and spitting
- Paper towels
- Physician's names and phone numbers
- "Thank you for being patient" yikes cards
- Urinal for men, prior to incontinence
- Waterproof seat pads, full-length, twin-bed size
- Wet wipes
- Disposable gloves
- Change of clothes

Caregiver Grief Inventory Form

MM Caregiver Grief Inventory	Thomas M. Meuser, Ph.D., Washington University, St. Louis Samuel J. Marwit, Ph.D., University of Missouri-St. Louis

Instructions: This inventory is designed to measure the grief experience of current family caregivers of persons living with progressive dementia (e.g., Alzheimer's disease). Read each statement carefully, then decide how much you agree or disagree with what is said. Circle a number 1-5 to the right using the answer key below (For example 5 = Strongly Agree). It is important that you respond to all items so that the scores are accurate. Scoring rules are listed at the end.

ANSWER KEY
1 = Strongly Disagree   // 2 = Disagree   // 3 = Somewhat Agree   // 4 = Agree   // 5 = Strongly Agree

#	Statement	1	2	3	4	5	
1	I've had to give up a great deal to be a caregiver.	1	2	3	4	5	A
2	I miss so many of the activities we used to share.	1	2	3	4	5	B
3	I feel I am losing my freedom.	1	2	3	4	5	A
4	My physical health has declined from the stress of being a caregiver.	1	2	3	4	5	A
5	I have nobody to communicate with.	1	2	3	4	5	C
6	I don't know what is happening. I feel confused and unsure.	1	2	3	4	5	C
7	I carry a lot of stress as a caregiver.	1	2	3	4	5	A
8	I receive enough emotional support from others.	1	2	3	4	5	Cr
9	I have this empty, sick feeling knowing that my loved one is "gone".	1	2	3	4	5	B
10	I feel anxious and scared.	1	2	3	4	5	C
11	My personal life has changed a great deal.	1	2	3	4	5	A
12	I spend a lot of time worrying about the bad things to come.	1	2	3	4	5	C
13	Dementia is like a double loss...I've lost the closeness with my loved one and connectedness with my family.	1	2	3	4	5	C
14	I feel terrific sadness	1	2	3	4	5	B
15	This situation is totally unacceptable in my heart.	1	2	3	4	5	B
16	My friends simply don't understand what I'm going through.	1	2	3	4	5	C
17	I feel this constant sense of responsibility and it just never leaves.	1	2	3	4	5	A
18	I long for what was, what we had and shared in the past.	1	2	3	4	5	B
19	I could deal with other serious disabilities better than with this.	1	2	3	4	5	B
20	I can't feel free in this situation.	1	2	3	4	5	A
21	I'm having trouble sleeping.	1	2	3	4	5	A
22	I'm at peace with myself and my situation in life.	1	2	3	4	5	Cr
23	It's a life phase and I know we'll get through it.	1	2	3	4	5	Cr
24	My extended family has no idea what I go through in caring for him/her.	1	2	3	4	5	C
25	I feel so frustrated that I often tune him/her out.	1	2	3	4	5	A
26	I am always worrying.	1	2	3	4	5	C
27	I'm angry at the disease for robbing me of so much.	1	2	3	4	5	B
28	This is requiring more emotional energy and determination than I ever expected.	1	2	3	4	5	A
29	I will be tied up with this for who knows how long.	1	2	3	4	5	A
30	It hurts to put her/him to bed at night and realize that she/he is "gone"	1	2	3	4	5	B
31	I feel very sad about what this disease has done.	1	2	3	4	5	B
32	I feel severe depression.	1	2	3	4	5	C

	ANSWER KEY 1 = **Strongly Disagree** // 2 = Disagree // 3 = Somewhat Agree // 4 = Agree // 5 = **Strongly Agree**						
33	I lay awake most nights worrying about what's happening and how I'll manage tomorrow.	1	2	3	4	5	C
34	The people closest to me do not understand what I'm going through.	1	2	3	4	5	C
35	His/her death will bring me renewed personal freedom to live my life.	1	2	3	4	5	A
36	I feel powerless.	1	2	3	4	5	B
37	It's frightening because you know doctors can't cure this disease, so things only get worse.	1	2	3	4	5	B
38	I've lost other people close to me, but the losses I'm experiencing now are much more troubling.	1	2	3	4	5	B
39	Independence is what I've lost…I don't have the freedom to go and do what I want.	1	2	3	4	5	A
40	I've had to make some drastic changes in my life as a result of becoming a caregiver.	1	2	3	4	5	A
41	I wish I had an hour or two to myself each day to pursue personal interests.	1	2	3	4	5	A
42	I'm stuck in this caregiving world and there's nothing I can do about it.	1	2	3	4	5	A
43	I can't contain my sadness about all that's happening.	1	2	3	4	5	B
44	What upsets me most is what I've had to give up.	1	2	3	4	5	A
45	I'm managing pretty well overall.	1	2	3	4	5	Cr
46	I think I'm denying the full implications of this for my life.	1	2	3	4	5	C
47	I get excellent support from members of my family.	1	2	3	4	5	Cr
48	I've had a hard time accepting what is happening.	1	2	3	4	5	B
49	The demands on me are growing faster than I ever expected.	1	2	3	4	5	A
50	I wish this was all a dream and I could wake up back in my old life.	1	2	3	4	5	B

FAIR USE OF THE MM-CGI: The inventory was developed and pilot tested on two samples of dementia caregivers: 87 caregivers (45 adult child, 42 spouse) in the development phase and 166 (83 of each type) for pilot testing. Funding support came from the Alzheimer's Association (Grant 1999-PRG-1730). A 3-factor solution materialized (KMO = .889) and these factors are listed below. The authors consider this instrument to be part of the public domain. The authors would appreciate hearing feedback on how the scale is used. Researchers who wish to administer the inventory and/or modify it as part of a formal study are asked to notify the authors of their plans (Tom Meuser, Ph.D., meusert@umsl.edu; 314-516-5421).

Meuser, T.M., & Marwit, S.J. (2001). A comprehensive, stage-sensitive model of grief in dementia caregiving. The Gerontologist, Vol 41(5), 658-770.

Marwit, S.J., & Meuser, T.M. (2002). Development and Initial Validation of an Inventory to Assess Grief in Caregivers of Persons with Alzheimer's Disease. The Gerontologist, 42(6), 751-765.

Self-Scoring Procedure: Add the numbers you circled to derive the following sub-scale and total grief scores. Use the letters to the right of each score to guide you. *C Items with "r" afterwards must first be reverse scored (1→5, 2→4, 3→3, 4→2, 5→1) before adding to calculate your scores.*

Personal Sacrifice Burden *(A Items)* = _____
(18 Items, M = 54.3, SD = 14.1, Alpha = .93, Split-Half = .91)

Heartfelt Sadness & Longing *(B Items)* = _____
(15 Items, M = 48.2, SD = 11.1, Alpha = .90, Split-Half = .88)

Worry & Felt Isolation *(C Items)* = _____
(17 Items, M = 40.6, SD = 11.9, Alpha = .91, Split-Half = .91)

Total Grief Level (Sum A + B + C) = _____
(50 Items, M = 144, SD = 31.6, Alpha = .96, Split-Half = .87)

Plot your scores using the grid to the right. Make an "X" in the shaded section nearest to your numeric score for each sub-scale. This is your grief profile. Discuss this profile with your support group leader or counselor.

MM-CGI Personal Grief Profile

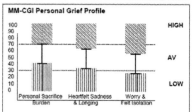

What do these scores mean?

Scores in the top area are higher than average based validation sample statistics (1 SD above the Mean). High scores may indicate a need for formal intervention or support assistance to enhance coping. Low scores in the bottom lined section (1 SD below the Mean) may indicate denial or a downplaying of distress. Low scores may also indicate positive adaptation if the individual is not showing other signs of suppressed grief. Average scores in the center indicate common reactions. These are general guides for discussion and support only – more research is needed on more specific interpretation issues.

MM Caregiver Grief Inventory is Public Domain

Checklist Following Death

☐ Call hospice, attending physician, or coroner to pronounce the patient's death

☐ If applicable, notify brain donation and/or autopsy research institution for instructions

☐ Inform immediate family members and close friends

☐ Call the funeral home to discuss burial arrangements

☐ Request 10-15 copies of the Death Certificate from your funeral director

☐ Prepare and arrange for the obituary

☐ Explore veteran's burial allowance and/or additional benefits

☐ Do not pay decedent's debts until you obtain the advice of an Attorney

☐ Notify your local Social Security office

☐ Contact the health insurance companies regarding coverage for the deceased

□ Contact the insurance company about life insurance policies. You will need to provide:
1. The policy number
2. A certified copy of the death certificate

□ Inform credit card companies of the decedent's death

□ Seek the advice of a CPA and/or attorney about filing the deceased's tax return for the year of the death. Keep monthly bank statements on all individual and joint accounts that show the account balance on the day of death. You will need this information for the estate tax return.

□ Change joint bank accounts into your name

□ Check with the bank for a safe deposit box

□ Locate wills and trusts

□ Transfer the car title into your name

□ Change stocks and bonds into your name. Contact your bank or stockbroker for the proper forms.

□ Obtain the value of all assets if needed

☐ Complete (with assistance if necessary) final income and estate tax returns

Additional documents that may be required to accomplish the above tasks:

- Automobile Title and Registration Papers
- Bank Books
- Birth Certificate
- Birth Certificate for each child, if applicable
- Death Certificates (10–15 certified copies)
- Deed and Titles to Property
- Discharge Papers for a Veteran and/or V.A. Claim Number
- Insurance Policies
- Loan and Installment Payment Books and/or Contracts
- Marriage Certificate
- Recent Income Tax Forms and W-2 Forms
- Social Security Card
- Stock Certificates

Clinical Dementia Rating Scale, aka CDR

		NONE 0	QUESTIONABLE 0.5	MILD 1	MODERATE 2	SEVERE 3
Memory		No memory loss or slight Inconsistent forgetfulness	Consistent slight forgetfulness; partial recollection of events; "benign" forgetfulness	Moderate memory loss: more marked for recent events; defect interferes with everyday activity	Severe memory loss; only highly learned material retained: new material rapidly lost	Severe memory loss; only fragments remain
Orientation		Fully oriented	Fully oriented but with slight difficulty with time relationships	Moderate difficulty with time relationships; oriented for place at examination; may have geographic disorientation elsewhere	Severe difficulty with time relationships; usually disoriented to time, often to place	Oriented to person only

Judgment and Problem-Solving	Solves everyday problems and handles business and financial affairs well; judgment good in relation to past performance	Slight impairment in solving problems, similarities and differences	Moderate difficulty in handling problems, similarities and differences; social judgment usually maintained	Severely impaired in handling problems, similarities and differences; social judgment usually impaired	Unable to make judgments or solve problems
Community Affairs	Independent function as usual in job, shopping, volunteer and social groups	Slight impairment in these activities	Unable to function independently at these activities, though may still be engaged in some; appears normal to casual inspection	No pretense of independent function home; appears well enough to be taken to functions outside the family home	Appears too ill to be taken to functions outside the family home

Home and Hobbies	Life at home, hobbies and intellectual interests well maintained	Life at home, hobbies and intellectual interests slightly impaired	Mild but definite impairment of functions at home; more difficult chores, and complicated hobbies and interests abandoned	Only simple chores preserved; very restricted interests, poorly maintained	No significant function in the home
Personal Care	Fully capable of self-care		Needs prompting	Requires assistance in dressing, hygiene, and keeping of personal effects	Requires much help with personal care; frequent incontinence

Cohen-Mansfield Agitation Inventory (CMAI)

The author advises consulting the manual prior to using the CMAI. The manual can be found on the following website:

http://www.dementia-assessment.com.au/symptoms/CMAI_Manual.pdf

Instructions: For each of the behaviors below, check the rating that indicates the average frequency of occurrence over the last 2 weeks.

Behavior	Never 1	Less Than Once a Week 2	Once or Twice a Week 3	Several Times a Week 4	Once or Twice a Day 5	Several Times a Day 6	Several Times an Hour 7
1. Hitting (including self)	❏	❏	❏	❏	❏	❏	❏
2. Kicking	❏	❏	❏	❏	❏	❏	❏
3. Grabbing onto people	❏	❏	❏	❏	❏	❏	❏
4. Pushing	❏	❏	❏	❏	❏	❏	❏
5. Throwing things	❏	❏	❏	❏	❏	❏	❏
6. Biting	❏	❏	❏	❏	❏	❏	❏
7. Scratching	❏	❏	❏	❏	❏	❏	❏
8. Spitting	❏	❏	❏	❏	❏	❏	❏
9. Hurt self or others	❏	❏	❏	❏	❏	❏	❏
10. Tearing things or destroying property	❏	❏	❏	❏	❏	❏	❏
11. Making physical sexual advances	❏	❏	❏	❏	❏	❏	❏
12. Paces, aimless wandering	❏	❏	❏	❏	❏	❏	❏
13. Inappropriate dress or disrobing	❏	❏	❏	❏	❏	❏	❏
14. Trying to get to a different place.	❏	❏	❏	❏	❏	❏	❏
15. Intentional falling	❏	❏	❏	❏	❏	❏	❏
16. Eating/drinking inappropriate substances	❏	❏	❏	❏	❏	❏	❏
17. Handling things inappropriately	❏	❏	❏	❏	❏	❏	❏
18. Hiding things	❏	❏	❏	❏	❏	❏	❏
19. Hoarding things	❏	❏	❏	❏	❏	❏	❏
20. Performing repetitious mannerisms	❏	❏	❏	❏	❏	❏	❏
21. General restlessness	❏	❏	❏	❏	❏	❏	❏
22. Screaming	❏	❏	❏	❏	❏	❏	❏
23. Making verbal sexual advances	❏	❏	❏	❏	❏	❏	❏
24. Cursing or verbal aggression	❏	❏	❏	❏	❏	❏	❏
25. Repetitive sentences or questions	❏	❏	❏	❏	❏	❏	❏
26. Strange noises (weird laughter or crying)	❏	❏	❏	❏	❏	❏	❏
27. Complaining	❏	❏	❏	❏	❏	❏	❏
28. Negativism	❏	❏	❏	❏	❏	❏	❏
29. Constant unwarranted request for attention or help	❏	❏	❏	❏	❏	❏	❏

Name of Rater:

Name of Primary Caregiver/Informant:

Note: This is the nursing-home, long version of the Cohen-Mansfield Agitation Inventory. For definitions of the behaviors, administration, scoring information, and other versions, please consult the manual.

Original article: Cohen-Mansfield, J., Marx, M. S., & Rosenthal, A. S. (1989). A description of agitation in a nursing home. *Journal of Gerontology: Medical Sciences*, 44(3), M77–M84.

Emergency Room Kit

- Current medications, dosage, and prescribing doctor
- List of known allergies
- Pharmacy phone numbers
- Diagnosis on physician's letterhead
- Primary care doctor's name and phone number
- Neurologist's name and phone number
- Geriatric Psychiatrist's name and phone number
- Emergency names and phone numbers
- Copy of insurance cards
- Copy of legal guardianship/conservator papers
- Copy of Health Care Power of Attorney with HIPAA Release Authority
- Copy of Living Will
- Photo I.D./driver's license
- Caregivers' names and phone numbers
- Medical Release Form
- If desired, DNR (Do Not Resuscitate) order

Functional Assessment Staging Scale (FAST)

At the New York University Medical Center's Aging and Dementia Research Center, Barry Reisberg, MD and colleagues have developed the Functional Assessment Staging (FAST) scale, which allows professionals and caregivers to chart the decline of people with Alzheimer's disease. The FAST scale has 16 stages and sub-stages:

FAST Scale Stage	Characteristics
1... normal adult	No functional decline.
2... normal older adult	Personal awareness of some functional decline.
3... early Alzheimer's disease	Noticeable deficits in demanding job situations.
4... mild Alzheimer's	Requires assistance in complicated tasks such as handling finances, planning parties, etc.
5... moderate Alzheimer's	Requires assistance in choosing proper attire.
6... moderately severe Alzheimer's	Requires assistance dressing, bathing, and toileting. Experiences urinary and fecal incontinence.
7... severe Alzheimer's	Speech ability declines to about a half-dozen intelligible words. Progressive loss of abilities to walk, sit up, smile, and hold head up.

"I obtained a short version of the scale from my husbands' hospice caregiver."

Pain Assessment for Advanced/Non-verbal Dementia Patient (PAINAD) Scale

Pain Assessment in Advanced Dementia Scale (PAINAD)

Instructions: Observe the patient for five minutes before scoring his or her behaviors. Score the behaviors according to the following chart. Definitions of each item are provided on the following page. The patient can be observed under different conditions (e.g., at rest, during a pleasant activity, during caregiving, after the administration of pain medication).

Behavior	0	1	2	Score
Breathing Independent of vocalization	• Normal	• Occasional labored breathing • Short period of hyperventilation	• Noisy labored breathing • Long period of hyperventilation • Cheyne-Stokes respirations	
Negative vocalization	• None	• Occasional moan or groan • Low-level speech with a negative or disapproving quality	• Repeated troubled calling out • Loud moaning or groaning • Crying	
Facial expression	• Smiling or inexpressive	• Sad • Frightened • Frown	• Facial grimacing	
Body language	• Relaxed	• Tense • Distressed pacing • Fidgeting	• Rigid • Fists clenched • Knees pulled up • Pulling or pushing away • Striking out	
Consolability	• No need to console	• Distracted or reassured by voice or touch	• Unable to console, distract, or reassure	
			TOTAL SCORE	

(Warden et al., 2003)

Scoring:

The total score ranges from 0-10 points. A possible interpretation of the scores is: 1-3=mild pain; 4-6=moderate pain; 7-10=severe pain. These ranges are based on a standard 0-10 scale of pain, but have not been substantiated in the literature for this tool.

Source:

Warden V, Hurley AC, Volicer L. Development and psychometric evaluation of the Pain Assessment in Advanced Dementia (PAINAD) scale. *J Am Med Dir Assoc.* 2003;4(1):9-15.

PAINAD Item Definitions
(Warden et al., 2003)

Breathing
1. *Normal breathing* is characterized by effortless, quiet, rhythmic (smooth) respirations.
2. *Occasional labored breathing* is characterized by episodic bursts of harsh, difficult, or wearing respirations.
3. *Short period of hyperventilation* is characterized by intervals of rapid, deep breaths lasting a short period of time.
4. *Noisy labored breathing* is characterized by negative-sounding respirations on inspiration or expiration. They may be loud, gurgling, wheezing. They appear strenuous or wearing.
5. *Long period of hyperventilation* is characterized by an excessive rate and depth of respirations lasting a considerable time.
6. *Cheyne-Stokes respirations* are characterized by rhythmic waxing and waning of breathing from very deep to shallow respirations with periods of apnea (cessation of breathing).

Negative Vocalization
1. *None* is characterized by speech or vocalization that has a neutral or pleasant quality.
2. *Occasional moan or groan* is characterized by mournful or murmuring sounds, wails, or laments. Groaning is characterized by louder than usual inarticulate involuntary sounds, often abruptly beginning and ending.
3. *Low level speech with a negative or disapproving quality* is characterized by muttering, mumbling, whining, grumbling, or swearing in a low volume with a complaining, sarcastic, or caustic tone.
4. *Repeated troubled calling out* is characterized by phrases or words being used over and over in a tone that suggests anxiety, uneasiness, or distress.
5. *Loud moaning or groaning* is characterized by mournful or murmuring sounds, wails, or laments in much louder than usual volume. Loud groaning is characterized by louder than usual inarticulate involuntary sounds, often abruptly beginning and ending.
6. *Crying* is characterized by an utterance of emotion accompanied by tears. There may be sobbing or quiet weeping.

Facial Expression
1. *Smiling or inexpressive.* Smiling is characterized by upturned corners of the mouth, brightening of the eyes, and a look of pleasure or contentment. Inexpressive refers to a neutral, at ease, relaxed, or blank look.
2. *Sad* is characterized by an unhappy, lonesome, sorrowful, or dejected look. There may be tears in the eyes.
3. *Frightened* is characterized by a look of fear, alarm, or heightened anxiety. Eyes appear wide open.
4. *Frown* is characterized by a downward turn of the corners of the mouth. Increased facial wrinkling in the forehead and around the mouth may appear.
5. *Facial grimacing* is characterized by a distorted, distressed look. The brow is more wrinkled, as is the area around the mouth. Eyes may be squeezed shut.

Body Language
1. *Relaxed* is characterized by a calm, restful, mellow appearance. The person seems to be taking it easy.
2. *Tense* is characterized by a strained, apprehensive, or worried appearance. The jaw may be clenched. (Exclude any contractures.)
3. *Distressed pacing* is characterized by activity that seems unsettled. There may be a fearful, worried, or disturbed element present. The rate may be faster or slower.
4. *Fidgeting* is characterized by restless movement. Squirming about or wiggling in the chair may occur. The person might be hitching a chair across the room. Repetitive touching, tugging, or rubbing body parts can also be observed.
5. *Rigid* is characterized by stiffening of the body. The arms and/or legs are tight and inflexible. The trunk may appear straight and unyielding. (Exclude any contractures.)
6. *Fists clenched* is characterized by tightly closed hands. They may be opened and closed repeatedly or held tightly shut.
7. *Knees pulled up* is characterized by flexing the legs and drawing the knees up toward the chest. An overall troubled appearance. (Exclude any contractures.)
8. *Pulling or pushing away* is characterized by resistiveness upon approach or to care. The person is trying to escape by yanking or wrenching him- or herself free or shoving you away.
9. *Striking out* is characterized by hitting, kicking, grabbing, punching, biting, or other form of personal assault.

Consolability
1. *No need to console* is characterized by a sense of well-being. The person appears content.
2. *Distracted or reassured by voice or touch* is characterized by a disruption in the behavior when the person is spoken to or touched. The behavior stops during the period of interaction, with no indication that the person is at all distressed.
3. *Unable to console, distract, or reassure* is characterized by the inability to soothe the person or stop a behavior with words or actions. No amount of comforting, verbal or physical, will alleviate the behavior.

Personal Portfolio

Portfolio Items	Location
Alarm system directions, phone numbers, and code	
Driver's license numbers	
Veteran's discharge papers	
Copy of marriage license	
Resumes	
Copy of birth certificates	
Social Security numbers	
Passports	
Emergency contacts and phone numbers	
Support groups and phone numbers	
Personal physicians and phone numbers	
Insurance policy and phone numbers	
Insurance policy: annual cost	
Insurance policy: date last paid	
Copy of Medicare and insurance card	
Monthly income	
Bank account numbers (checking/savings)	
Monthly expense spreadsheets	
Bank contact information	
Retirement account names/ numbers	
Financial consultant's contact information	

Safety deposit box/keys location; co-signer info if applicable	
House deeds	
Car titles	
VIN number	
License number	
Inventory of Collections	
Financial misc./other assets	
Properties/real estate deeds (ID #, estimated value, contacts)	
Superior Court Guardianship documents	
Living wills	
Wills	
Power of attorney, medical	
Power of attorney, financial	
Living trust	
Attorney contact information	

Sample Daily Journal

Sample Daily Journal	Date: _____
Medications	
Allergies	
Memory	
Daily Activities	
Behavior	
Appearance	
Eating Habits	
Food Cravings	
Sleep Routine	
Unusual Events	
Questions	

Sample Medical Release Form

(Your Name)
(Street Address)
(City, ST ZIP Code)

Date:

(Doctor Name)
(Medical Practice or Hospital Name)
(Street Address)
(City, ST ZIP Code)

RE: Authorization to release medical records for (patient's name)

DOB: (date of birth)

Dear (Doctor Name):
I am writing to authorize (Attorney Name or Advocate Name) to obtain medical records on (Patient's Name) behalf. Please release his/her medical records related to treatment for (medical condition(s)) rendered by you or under your supervision from (date) through (date).

If you have any questions, please call me at (your phone number) or (Attorney Name or Advocate Name) at (Attorney or Advocate phone number).

Sincerely,
(Your Name)
cc:

Sample Medication Chart

Monday

Medication	Dose time	Dose time	Dose time	Dose time	Dose time

Tuesday

Medication	Dose time	Dose time	Dose time	Dose time	Dose time

Wednesday

Medication	Dose time	Dose time	Dose time	Dose time	Dose time

Thursday

Medication	Dose time	Dose time	Dose time	Dose time	Dose time

Friday

Medication	Dose time	Dose time	Dose time	Dose time	Dose time

Saturday

Medication	Dose time	Dose time	Dose time	Dose time	Dose time

Sunday

Medication	Dose time	Dose time	Dose time	Dose time	Dose time

Sample Physician's Letter

Dr. John Doe
0000 Market Street
Broken Bone, NM
00000

Phone Number: 1-000-000-0000

Re: [Patient Name], Date of Birth:

To Whom It May Concern:

The above-named patient has a progressive, degenerative disorder of his central nervous system. He/She shows difficulties in memory, language skills, and cognition. This has been demonstrated by a neuropsychologist as well as neurologist, [Doctor's name], at [facility].

It is in the best interest of all that my patient not fly a plane, drive, or make financial or life-altering decisions.

Please feel free to contact me regarding any further information concerning this matter.

Sincerely,

John Doe, M.D.

ADULT DAYCARE
Eldercare Locator
The service is provided by the United States Administration on Aging. The website allows you to obtain information and assistance for the elderly by topic, location, or zip code. They offer resources and links for almost any subject matter.

Toll-Free Phone Number: 1-800-677-1116

Available Weekdays, 9:00 a.m. to 8:00 p.m. (ET).

http://www.eldercare.gov/eldercare.net/Public

ADVANCE DIRECTIVES
Aging with Dignity
For a small fee you can purchase **Five Wishes, a do-it-yourself advance directive.** It is considered a legal document in all but eight states.

Five Wishes—A do-it-yourself advance directive

Toll-Free Phone Number: 888-5WISHES (594-7437)

http://www.agingwithdignity.org/five-wishes.php

Caring Connections

This website provides free printable advance directive downloads and instructions by state, in PDF file format.

http://www.caringinfo.org/stateaddownload

BOOKS

Interactive Therapeutics, now part of AliMed Products

"AliMed offers a variety of health care books and speech products designed to help caregivers communicate with patients with language deficits by means of pictures and/or words."

Toll-Free Phone Number: 1-800-225-2610

http://www.alimed.com/Alimed/catalog/Interactive-Therapeutic,339.htm

The 36-Hour Day: A Family Guide to Caring for Persons With Alzheimer's Disease, Related Dementing Illnesses, and Memory Loss in Later Life.

Nancy L. Mace, M.A., and Peter V. Rabins, M.D., M.P.H.

The Dysphagia Cookbook

Elayne Achilles

Today's Caregiver Magazine

The magazine, as well as the website, offers information, resources, support, and guidance to caregivers and families.

Toll-Free Phone Number: 1-800-829-2734

http://www.caregiver.com/magazine

BRAIN DONATION

Boston University School of Medicine's Alzheimer's Disease Center

Toll-Free Phone Number: 1-888-458-2823

http://www.bu.edu/alzresearch/research/memory/hope/brain.html

Butler Hospital Memory & Aging Program

Phone Number: 1-401-455-6402

http://www.memorydisorder.org/braindonation.htm

Emory Alzheimer's Disease Research Center

For Clinic Appointment: Phone Number: 1-404-778-3444

To Volunteer for a Research Study:

Phone Number: 1-404-728-6950

http://med.emory.edu/ADRC

Northwestern University in Chicago

Phone Number: 1-312-695-2343 between 8:00 a.m. and 5:00 p.m., Monday through Friday
http://www.brain.northwestern.edu/mdad/brainendowment.html

University of California, San Francisco

This website offers numerous nationwide brain research and donation resources.
http://www.memory.ucsf.edu/Research/autopsy.html

University of Pennsylvania

The Brain Behavior Center of the University of Pennsylvania accepts brain and tissue donations from patients who live within a three-hour drive of Philadelphia.
Kevin Davies, Administrative Coordinator
Center for Neurodegenerative Disease Research
Phone Number: 1-215-662-4474
daviesk@mail.med.upenn.edu
http://www.med.upenn.edu/bbl/programs/donation

CAREGIVING
AARP
Foundation Programs offers an excellent "Planning Guide for Families."
http://assets.aarp.org/www.aarp.org_/articles/foundation/aa66r2_care.pdf

To obtain a copy of "A Planning Guide For Adult Care" call the phone number below.
Toll-Free Phone Number: 1-888-687-2277, Monday-Friday, 7:00 a.m.–midnight ET
Write: AARP Foundation Programs, 601 E Street NW, Washington, DC 20049

AGIS Network
AGIS specializes in elder care and long-term care products and services, including:
- Assisted Daily Living Aids
- Support Services
- Checklists & Assessments
- Find Local Services
- Home Care Support Services
- Home Safety and Improvement
- Help for Family Caregivers
- Free Caregiving Kit

Toll-Free Phone Number: 1-866-511-9186
http://www.agis.com

ARCH National Respite Network

The National Respite Locator Service helps to locate respite care services in your community.

Toll-Free Phone Number: 1-800-773-5433

http://www.respitelocator.org

Caring For Your Parents

This organization offers a free care guide, resources, and support to dementia caregivers.

Caring.com offers advice on money and legal matters, in-home care, senior living resources, caregiver wellness, and much more. This is a site worth exploring.

http://www.caring.com

Full Circle of Care

Full Circle of Care provides nationwide access to a multitude of caregiver services to support your efforts to keep your family member living at home.

http://www.fullcirclecare.org

Medicare.gov/caregivers

This is a United States government site for medicare support and assistance to caregivers of a seriously ill or disabled person.

http://www.medicare.gov/caregivers

National Association of Area Agencies on Aging

Their mission is to "help older persons and persons with disabilities live with dignity and choices in their homes and communities for as long as possible."

Years ago, thanks to government funding, I only paid pennies on the dollar for in-home assistance that they recommended. You should be able to find your local chapter of Area Agency on Aging in the phonebook.

Call: 1-202-872-8888

http://www.n4a.org

National Family Caregivers Association (NFCA)

I believe this Association is the ultimate caregiver advocate. They instruct, assist, empower, and speak up for caregivers of America.

Toll-Free Phone Number: 1-888-687-2277, Monday–Friday, 7:00 a.m.–midnight ET

Write: 10400 Connecticut Avenue, Suite 500, Kensington, MD 20895-3944

http://www.nfcacares.org

http://www.thefamilycaregiver.org/ed/resources.cfm

Yahoo! Support Groups

Create or join an online support group.

http://groups.yahoo.com

CLINICAL TRIALS

ClinicalTrials.gov

They have a nationwide database with current clinical research studies. You can search by the name, the medical condition, as well as by your location.

"Information on Clinical Trials and Human Research Studies."

http://www.ClinicalTrials.gov

National Institute on Aging

Search a database of clinical trials currently in progress at sites throughout the United States.
http://www.nia.nih.gov/Alzheimers/ResearchInformation/ClinicalTrials

CLOTHING

Silverts

"Disabled Adaptive Clothing, Senior Elderly Care Clothing, Shoes & Slippers"
Toll-Free Phone Number: 1-800-387-7088
http://www.silverts.com

DIAGNOSIS AND TREATMENT

Columbia Presbyterian Medical Center

Lucy G. Moses Center for Memory and Behavioral Disorders
New York, NY
Phone Number: 1-212-305-6939

Indiana University School of Medicine

Indiana Alzheimer's Disease Center
Indianapolis, IN
Phone Number: 1-317-278-5500

Johns Hopkins University School of Medicine
Frontotemporal Dementia and Young-Onset Dementias Clinic
Baltimore, MD
Phone Number: 1-410-502-2981

Northwestern University Feinberg School of Medicine Cognitive Neurology and Alzheimer's Disease Center
Chicago, IL
Phone Number: 1-312-908-9339
http://www.brain.northwestern.edu

The Association For Frontotemporal Dementias
Toll-Free Phone Number: 1-866-507-7222
http://ftd-picks.org

University of California, Los Angeles
Frontotemporal Dementia & Neurobehavior Clinic
Los Angeles, CA
Phone Number: 1-310-794-2550

University of California, San Francisco Memory and Aging Center

Phone Number: 1-415-476-6880 (main phone)

Fax: 1-415-476-4800

http://memory.ucsf.edu

University of Pennsylvania Health System

Center for Frontotemporal Dementia

Philadelphia, PA

Phone Number: 1-215-662-3606

DRUG INTERACTIONS

Medscape.com

This site allows you to check possible interactions between two or more drugs.

http://reference.medscape.com/drug-interaction-checker

DRUG ASSISTANCE PROGRAMS

Benefits Checkup Rx

Apply to qualify for Medicare Savings Programs to help pay for prescription drugs, health care, rent, utilities, and other fundamental needs.

http://www.benefitscheckup.org

Together Rx Access

"Ten leading pharmaceutical companies partnered together to provide a drug card program that will offer discounts on prescription drug purchases for uninsured Americans."

Toll-Free Phone Number: 1-800-444-4106

http://www.togetherrxaccess.com

Needymeds.com

If you qualify, this organization provides assistance to people who are unable to afford their medications, health care costs, and much more. Search for drug assistance programs by drug name or by pharmaceutical company/program.

http://www.needymeds.com

Partnership for Prescription Assistance

They will assist qualified patients without prescription drug coverage get the medicines they need.

Toll-Free Phone Number: 1-888-477-2669

http://www.pparx.org

FINANCIAL EMERGENCIES
Angel Food Ministries
This is a non-profit organization that buys food directly from suppliers at substantial volume discounts, passing the savings on to you.
Toll-Free Phone Number: 1-877-FOOD-MINISTRY
http://www.angelfoodministries.com

FINANCIAL AID AND CARE
The American Elder Care Research Organization
They offer financial options, aid, and locator caregiving resources for long-term care.
736 Cole Street
San Francisco, California 94117
Phone Number: 641-715-3900 Ext. 606151
http://www.payingforseniorcare.com/longtermcare/resources/locator_tool.html

HOME AIDE AND CAREGIVING RESOURCES
Alzheimer's Association's Respite Care Guide
Print a booklet to help research respite care available in your area.
http://www.alz.org/documents/Pub_respitecare-guide.pdf

NFCA
The National Family Caregivers Association
Free Family Caregiver Toolkit and Planner
Toll-Free Phone Number: 1-800-896-3650
http://www.thefamilycaregiver.org

Personal Care Finder
The Alzheimer's Association offers a personal care finder. After you enter your data, you can print your personalized information sheet. Speak to your patient's physician to help with any unanswered questions in regards to your loved one's condition and care options.
24/7 Helpline: 1-800-272-3900
http://www.alz.org/carefinder/careoptions/carenav1.asp

HOSPITALS
US News and World Report
Best Hospitals
This is an up-to-date website that provides a personalized hospital search to find the best hospital close to your location by specialty.
http://health.usnews.com/best-hospitals

INCONTINENCE AND DEMENTIA SUPPLIES

Comfort Plus Products

They provide an incontinence need and assessment selection guide to fit your specific incontinence needs.
Toll-Free Phone Number: 1-888-656-8055
http://www.comfortplusonline.com

Disposable Medical Express

Toll-Free Phone Number: 1-800-592-2848
http://www.disposablemedicalexpress.com

The Alzheimer's Store

The Alzheimer's Store offers almost any product you might need for dementia patients.
Toll-Free Phone Number: 1-800-752-3238
Fax: 1-678-947-8411
http://www.alzstore.com

The Bed Wetting Store

I purchased many of my waterproof washable mattress overlay pads from this site.
Toll-Free Phone Number: 1-800-214-9605
http://www.bedwettingstore.com

Tranquility Products

My personal favorite offers a complete line of adult disposable incontinence products.

Personal Use Questions

Toll-Free Phone Number: 1-800-467-3224, option 7

General Help

Toll-Free Phone Number: 1-800-467-3224, option 0

http://www.tranquilityproducts.com

MEDICATION

Medisave Canada

This discount, online pharmacy is located in Canada. For years I ordered our expensive medications from them. Our primary care doctor initially recommended them to me. I saved hundreds of dollars with every order.

http://www.medisave.ca/howtoorder.aspx

National Institute on Aging
Alzheimer's Disease Education and Referral (ADEAR) Center

Find out which prescription drugs are currently approved by the US Food and Drug Administration (FDA) to treat people who have been diagnosed with dementia. They offer a printable medication fact sheet.

Toll-Free Phone Number: 1-800-438-4380

http://www.nia.nih.gov/Alzheimers/Publications/medicationsfs.htm or

http://www.nia.nih.gov/Alzheimers

The Alzheimer's Association

This site "provides a list of non-drug approaches and treatments for cognitive, behavioral, and psychiatric symptoms."

http://www.alz.org/alzheimers_disease_standard_prescriptions.asp

Universal Drug Store

This is a licensed Canadian pharmacy that provides approved drugs at discounted prices.

Toll-Free Phone Number: 1-866-456-2456

Fax: 1-866-783-4223

http://www.universaldrugstore.com

University of San Francisco

UCSF provides up-to-date information on Alzheimer's and dementia medication.

http://memory.ucsf.edu/ftd/medical/treatment/avoid/multiple/benzodazepines

PHYSICIANS

American Medical Directors Association

"A national organization of long-term care physicians and members of the interdisciplinary team committed to quality care—the best resource for information to help care for your long-term care patients."

Toll-Free Phone Number: 1-800-876-2632

http://www.amda.com/contact.cfm

PLACEMENT AND LONG-TERM CARE

AGIS

AssistGuide Information Services

Alzheimer's and Dementia Facility Checklists

Toll-Free Phone Number: 1-866-511-9186

http://www.agis.com

A Place for Mom

Search for Senior Care by State.

http://www.aplaceformom.com

Geri Hall

Geri Hall has led the way in care strategies for people with Alzheimer's disease and related dementias. Her publications are currently available through the University Of Iowa Center on Aging, and well worth reading when faced with a placement concern.

Please read: *Helping Your Elder Adjust to a Residential Facility.*

http://www.ec-online.net/Knowledge/articles/adjusting.html

SAFETY
AGIS

Home safety for people with Alzheimer's disease.

Toll-Free Phone Number: 1-866-511-9186

http://www.agis.com

Alzheimer's Association

Contact them to request a free home safety brochure.

Safety Center 24/7 Toll-Free Helpline: 1-800-272-3900

http://www.alz.org/national/documents/brochure_homesafety.pdf or

http://www.alz.org/safetycenter/we_can_help_safety_issues.asp

Alzheimer's Disease Education and Referral (ADEAR) Center

Free home-safety brochure.

Toll-Free Phone Number: 1-800-438-4380

http://www.nia.nih.gov/Alzheimers

Everyday Health

Home safety information.

http://www.everydayhealth.com/alzheimers/alzheimers-care-home-safety.aspx

Medic Alert/Safe Return program

This is a "24-hour emergency response service for individuals with Alzheimer's or a related dementia, that wanders or has a medical emergency."

Toll-Free Phone Number: 1-888-633-4298

Enroll online: http://www.medicalert.org

National Institute on Aging

http://www.nia.nih.gov/Alzheimers/Publications/homesafety.htm

This Caring Home

http://www.thiscaringhome.org

UСan Health LLC

UCan Health sells a large variety of patient alarms.

Toll-Free Phone Number: 1-866-880-8226

Fax: 425-654-2322

http://ucanhealth.com/patient_alarm.htm

SOCIAL SECURITY ADMINISTRATION

Social Security Compassionate Allowances Program

This site lists up-to-date allowance medical conditions and provides information about how to apply. Applying for this program will speed up the process of disability claims for applicants with specific serious medical conditions.

Toll-Free Phone Number: 1-800-772-1213

http://www.socialsecurity.gov/compassionateallowances

Social Security Disability

Toll-Free Phone Number: 1-800-772-1213

http://www.ssa.gov/disability

Veterans Administration

Toll-Free Phone Number: 1-800-827-1000

http://www.va.gov/health

REFERENCES

- AARP
- http://www.aarp.org/magazine
- Alzheimer's Association
- Alzheimer's Disease Education and Referral (ADEAR) Center
- Alzheimer's Safe Return
- http://alzheimers.org.uk
- Andrea Petersen, Wall Street Journal, August 26, 2004
- Bradley R. Williams, PharmD, FASCP, CBP
- Careguide.com
- Center, University of Southern California
- Drugdigest.org
- Family Caregiver Alliance (FCA)
- Full Circle of Care
- Global Action on Aging
- Healthline.com
- Hospice of the Valley, Phoenix, Arizona
- http://www.peacehealth.org
- MedicineNet.com
- National Caregivers Association
- National Hospice and Palliative Care Organization
- National Institute on Aging

- New York University Medical Center's Aging and Dementia Research Center
- Ethel Perscy Andrus, Professor, Clinical Pharmacy & Clinical Gerontology, School of Pharmacy
- The Everett Clinic
- The Fisher Center for Alzheimer's Research Foundation
- The National Institute of Neurological Disorders and Stroke
- The National Institute on Aging
- http://www.Wikipedia.org/wiki/Veterans_benefits

INDEX